ANTI-AGING
THE CURE

ANTI-AGING
THE CURE
Based on Your Body Type

Manon Pilon

Sgräff

PO.Box 155, Station Place d'Armes, Montréal, Canada, H2Y 3E9

Library and Archives Canada Cataloguing in Publication

Pilon, Manon, 1965-

    Anti-aging : the cure based on your body type

    Includes bibliographical references.

    ISBN 2-923503-01-5

      1. Rejuvenation. 2. Aging - Prevention. 3. Health behavior. 4. Somatotypes. I. Title.

RA776.75.P5413 2006   613'.0434   C2006-940010-5

Legal Deposit:
National Library of Canada
Bibliothèque nationale du Québec

Research and interviews: Bernard Dubreuil
Editorial services and revision: Tina Anderes, Keren Penney and Science Communications Group
Illustrations: Dolphin Studios
Graphic design and page layout: Derome design

Printed in Canada by Interglobe

©Sgräff, 2006
http://www.sgraff.com

ISBN: 2-923503-01-5

1 2 3 4 5 09 08 07 06

"Manon Pilon is an internationally acclaimed anti-aging expert. She is a charismatic, passionate and inspiring keynote speaker. Manon's expertise is sought after around the world by doctors, estheticians, skin specialists and other players in the anti-aging field."

Dr. Robert Goldman, Chairman of the Board-American Academy of Anti-Aging Medicine (A4M)
Chairman of the Board-IFBB International Sportsmedicine Medical Commission (176 nations)

"If Hippocrates is considered the father of medicine, Manon Pilon is the sister to medical aesthetics!"

Lisa Lasher, OB/GYN, Medical Spa, Kentucky

"This book will teach you to age gracefully. Thanks to its clarity and depth, Manon Pilon's work is simply outstanding.

Michel Delune, M.D., President of the American Academy of Aesthetic Medicine (AAAM)

"I am honored to endorse Manon Pilon. My staff and I use her valuable principles and techniques in my dermatology practice, with outstanding results."

William P. Baugh, Medical Director, Full Spectrum Dermatology

"It is increasingly uncommon these days to find a skin care educator who is not only extremely knowledgeable but also highly professional, attractive, and well spoken. Manon Pilon is all of these and more. The concepts and techniques she teaches are based upon medical science and greater than twenty years of clinical experience. I am pleased to fully endorse her as a person, educator, and provider of skin health and beauty."

William P.Baugh, Medical Director, Full Spectrum Dermatology

"Manon Pilon has helped thousands of people become aware of their body type. By doing this, they have been able to make more informed decisions about their well-being."

Derrick M. DeSilva, Jr., M.D., Medical Director of the Medical Day Spa Association

"Manon Pilon's knowledge of skin and skin disorders, with her methods of communication, allowed our patients to understand better the overall aging of the skin."

Arie Benchetrit, FRCS(C), Plastic Surgeon, Cosmedica, Montreal

Manon Pilon

Manon Pilon is an internationally renowned authority on beauty and a leading world expert on morphology.

She is a passionate keynote speaker and has been invited all over the globe to share her secrets and knowledge acquired over decades of extensive research. A frequent guest speaker at several medical conferences, including A4M (American Academy on Anti-Aging Medicine), the Pan American College of Aesthetic Medicine, and the American Academy of Aesthetic Medicine, Manon Pilon has also addressed Les Nouvelles Esthetiques in Miami and in Paris; the Medical-Spa Conference; the International Spa Association (ISPA); the American Academy of Dermatology; the Spa and Resort Expo and the Medical Spa Expo and Conference; was honorary speaker and president of one of the foremost Canadian conferences, the Esthetique Spa International, in Montreal, and has given talks in Toronto, Vancouver and New York; and hosted the International Asthetics Cosmetic and Spa Conference in Las Vegas and Orlando. She has been met with great acclaim at the largest aesthetic shows in North America.

Throughout her 22-year practice, Manon Pilon has kept abreast of the latest research, developments and strategies in the field of skincare, health and human relations. She founded her own private school of aesthetics in Quebec. She owns skincare distribution, development and production companies, which have created many jobs in the field, and has always encouraged ownership opportunities for her employees.

She has been honored on numerous occasions by different business and professional associations: she has been nominated by the National Bank of Canada for her achievements and has been recognized by the American Academy of Aesthetic Medicine, by several universities around the world, for her accomplishments.

She has appeared on several television shows in her capacities both as an esthetician and also as an entrepreneur. She has been an invited guest on radio talk shows, and has written articles for well-known trade and consumer magazines. *Anti-aging. The Cure Based on Your Body Type* is the first book in a series, which addresses every aspect of aging. It is elegantly written with clarity and balance.

Table of contents

Detailed morphological evaluation

The cure

Conclusion: learn, take preventive action, maintain equilibrium

Glossary

I dedicate this book to Francesco Calato, founder of Méthode Physiodermie and my inspiration in the field of morphology.

Disclaimer

The opinions and knowledge expressed in this book are those of the author at the time of publication. It was written as an informative text on the subject. Neither the author nor the publisher claim, in any way, to offer a diagnosis of, or medical treatment for, your condition. Nothing can replace a competent doctor's careful examination, expertise and attentive care. The author and the publisher decline all responsibility with regard to any health risks that you might encounter, directly or indirectly, through following the ideas expressed herein. Naturally, before putting any of the ideas in this book into effect, you are strongly advised to consult a doctor.

Introduction

You will be embarking on an amazing adventure as you read this book. You will learn how to identify your body type and how to cope gracefully with the effects of time. You will even learn ways of preserving your youthful looks and vigor!

A quick glance at the huge number of books on diet, beauty and interpersonal relationships soon shows that very few ask the fundamental question, "Who are you?"

Yet we know, intuitively, that we are all different! This is simply common sense. Rejuvenation treatments that work for some can be completely ineffective, or even dangerous, for others. Genetic makeup varies considerably from one person to another. Universal anti-aging remedies are an illusion, and any anti-aging treatment that is based on the idea that we are all alike is doomed to fail.

One key notion and statement

The key notion that forms the basis of this book is: people are all different. Why is it that (let us call him) John eats constantly but seems to burn calories, never putting on any weight? Why does Jane, who never exercises, still manage, at 50, to have the body of a teenager? Why do not the same causes always have the same effects?

The key notion that forms the basis of this book is: people are all different.

It is quite simple: men's and women's bodies fall into four main types, which stem from our genetic inheritance. The genetic mixes that occur from generation to generation mean that we have a dominant type in our makeup, along with traits that are characteristic of another type. This is why the same causes can have quite different effects on different body types.

The book also states a fact: even if we accept that we differ from our neighbors, most of us have no idea how or why these differences exist. The answer is to be found in history.

Several decades ago, modern medicine moved away from this age-old knowledge. Yet, for over two thousand years, practitioners of Indian, Chinese and Greco-Roman medicine had always sought to determine patient types. Before any diagnosis of illness was made, before suggesting any path of action, they studied the dominant physical and psychological traits that characterized the patient. Well before the birth of genetics, these ancient healers knew the difference between what is innate and what is acquired, between genotype and phenotype, between:

* What each of us inherits from our parents, and
* What each of us makes of our life

These differences are of far more importance than any differences in skin color or sex. In fact, these three traditional medicines refer as much to women as to men, to children as to adults, taking no account of ethnic origin. The logic behind the three, four, or five types that each identified can be applied just as well to women as to men, and as much to Chinese as to Africans.

Today, this holistic approach has disappeared in America, Europe and other western countries. The subject is never broached in public schools. Our modern medicine seems to be in a period we might call the Age of Medication. Research efforts are all geared towards finding drugs to alleviate the symptoms that bring patients to see their doctors, i.e., pain, inflammation and infection. Drugs combat specific illnesses with specific molecules, in the assumption that everyone reacts to the same medicine in the same way.

The next time you leave the doctor's office with a handful of pills, take a close look at the kind of person you are. What kind of life do you lead? Do you eat well? Do you sleep well? Do you take the time to smell the flowers? Do you exercise regularly? Do you drink lots of water? Do you take dietary supplements? Do you listen to your body? Is your head constantly crammed with worries? Do you have time to switch off? Do you have hobbies? Are you happy at work? Do you have a fulfilling relationship with your spouse? What do you do to relax? How do you make time for yourself? Do you feel in control of your life?

Generally, modern medicine does not worry itself with such questions. Doctors rarely try to find the reasons for the imbalance in people's lives, nor do they examine the values that motivate choices or try to find out what makes their patients tick. They are seldom interested in what their patients know or the resources they have at hand. In short, a diagnosis is made without ever assessing a patient's strengths and weaknesses.

Time and resources are short and today's medical practitioners rarely think about actively involving their patients. Most do not point out how patients can concretely contribute to their own healing process, to their weight-loss program, or to their rejuvenation treatment. Patients are therefore unaware of the advantages to be gained by becoming personally involved in their own health. Preventive education is delegated to third parties and ends ups fading into oblivion.

It is very important to realize that prevention is not just a matter of encouraging people to go for frequent check-ups for known diseases. Prevention means analyzing an individual as a whole, identifying strengths and weaknesses, and looking at values and lifestyle, well before any signs or symptoms of illness appear.

A question of culture

Techno-science has given physicians a veritable arsenal of diagnostic and therapeutic tools. These have allowed us to save lives and eradicate illness, and we have made a major leap in our understanding of the human body. Yet, in the wake of these extraordinary advances, doctors have gradually abandoned diagnostic methods that they find less precise and have put their trust in technology. They have therefore traded their careful, detailed observations for laboratory tests. Investigation is now carried out without the patient being present, and often in the absence of the doctor, too. Not to mention cures that, beyond taking medicine, do not involve the "patient" at all. Neither the patient nor the doctor is at the heart of the process today. We might even change the definition of medicine; it no longer falls into the realm of gentle healing art, but has joined the ranks of pure science.

Today we have scans and other wonders of modern technology that allow us to see absolutely everything inside the body; it remains true, though, that nothing can ever replace the practiced eye of an experienced practitioner.

The good old family doctor at the beginning of the 20th century could rely only on his stethoscope and his sharp eye. Like him, I base my approach on rigorous observation of the individual, considering the complete entity that makes up a person.

Human beings possess an innate and wonderful ability to ensure their health and longevity.

My point of departure is the belief that human beings possess an innate and wonderful ability to ensure their health and longevity. I am convinced that a person must be actively involved in his or her own recovery.

Although this ability can vary from one person to another, every human being possesses it. When people sign on to something that suits them, nothing can stand in their way. When a plan of treatment is especially adapted to the individual, improvements are seen at every level—muscles, bones, skin, mind, emotions and relationships within the family and at work. The whole self is involved, with every system contributing to re-establish an equilibrium.

Studies have shown just how important it is for people to take an active interest in life if they want to stay young and in good health. We have often observed that when people engage in activities that suit them as individuals, they are able to prolong their physical, intellectual and emotion health far beyond their expectations. They will appear youthful in everything they do.

Our challenge lies in pinpointing what it is that suits us.

First, we have to identify who we are.

Our challenge lies in pinpointing what it is that suits us. By this, I mean identifying what suits us personally rather than what suits the other people around us. First, we have to identify who we are. This is the first and the most important question: "What's my type?" Only when we have found the answer to this can we move on and consider the next questions: "Now that I know what type I am, how do I begin my rejuvenation process?" "What's the right treatment for me?"

In the first section of the book, I am going to describe the four principal dominant types and the two main morphological groups that categorize human beings. You will need to familiarize yourself with each type. In the second section, you will read about the different possibilities each person can explore according to his or her body type. As an illustration of the rejuvenation system that I have developed, I have interspersed descriptions of real cases and their results throughout this section.

At various points in the book, I have included exercises that are designed to help you develop and practice your perceptive skills. All of these are based on the method that I use myself for personal evaluations (see Detailed morphological evaluation). You will find them fun to do, but more importantly, they are absolutely necessary for honing your sense of observation to enable you to do a full evaluation.

If you are really curious and just cannot wait to get an idea of your dominant type, go through the quick questionnaires, which you will find in each section, to determine your type. But I do encourage you to learn to observe other people first. With the help of the exercises and through actually trying out the evaluation tests, you will find yourself better positioned to carry out your own self-diagnosis from a more neutral standpoint. Once you have finished your reading, it is a good idea to do a re-evaluation of your own characteristics.

Finally, I invite you to visit the following sites regularly for the latest information and advice on anti-aging: <antiagingthecure.com> and <manonpilon.com>

Is knowing what best suits us enough to ensure that we do what is best?

If I ask you, "Do you want to look younger?" you are probably going to answer yes. But, what if I ask, "Are you prepared to do what it takes to look younger?" I might hear you answer, "It depends..." So what is the hesitation about?

We are very good at setting new goals, but we are also very good at finding excuses for not seeing things through.

Perhaps it is lack of time or money, not enough willpower, not trusting the advice we are given, lack of self-confidence, or not really wanting to change. And so often we fall back on the vague, "Well, my doctor hasn't recommended it..." or "It hasn't been proven..."

When it comes down to it, finding reasons to refuse to change is always a lot easier than committing to change. We are all alike in this respect: passivity is in our nature. Old habits sit comfortably, and changing direction seems to demand a much greater effort than continuing on the same old path.

And, quite rightly, we wonder if it is worth the effort. We know exactly what we have now, but the fact is that we can never be sure about the future.

Even when we know full well what we should do, most of the time we do not do it, or we start but do not keep it up. We do not persevere. We would rather leave things as they are, waiting to see if they become more urgent, by which time they will demand our full attention. Even when we hear alarm bells ringing, we turn a deaf ear.

All this is quite normal. Making reasoned choices based on an in-depth knowledge of ourselves is not an easy thing. How easy is it to give clear answers to questions like, "What makes me tick? What makes me get up in the morning? What is it that makes me say one thing and not another?" Most of the time, our motives are unclear, complex and often contradictory. Most of us will admit that we act without really being aware of our inner-most intentions.

Where's the proof?

As you read this, you may well be thinking, "If this anti-aging cure is as effective as you say, then everyone would be talking about it! People would already be doing it!" Well, they are!

The best proof I can offer is to tell you about the 5,000 clients that have passed through my doors in the last 10 years.

My proof is the last 20 years that I have spent helping people who have come asking, "What can I do?" These people have spent long months and years looking for answers to their problems of wrinkles or pigmentation spots, of acne that refuses to respond to treatment, of being overweight despite every diet possible, of cellulite that persists no matter what they do, of irritable bowel syndrome that will not respond to medication, or of stress at work or at home. These are some of the testimonials I have accumulated over the course of my practice.

For the first time, through this book, my approach, method and experience are being made known to a wider audience.

What are the principles behind my approach?

Three principles govern my approach:
1 The anti-aging cure is **holistic**: it takes into account a person's body, mind and emotions.
2 The anti-aging cure is **personalized**: it is adapted to each person's lifestyle and body type.

3 The anti-aging cure is **coherent**: all advice and treatments are interrelated. They are designed to be in synergy with each other.

My approach is founded on two types of procedures:

1 My anti-aging cure starts with a precise, meticulous, evaluation, to gather as much detailed information as possible, which enables me to:
  - Identify the morphological group to which the person belongs: ample or angular;
  - Identify the person's morphological type: *red oval, green square, yellow rectangle, or white circle;*
  - Identify the person's coloring to discover the underlying temperament;
  - Assess a person's present state of health, discover any past health problems and eliminate the possibility of contra-indications;
  - Assess a person's lifestyle habits with regard to exercise, diet, skincare, inter-personal relationships and stress.

2 My anti-aging cure gives you both advice and treatment:
  - Advice on prevention and maintenance for those who are in generally good health and want to stay that way;
  - Advice on suitable remedies for those who show signs of aging or have a health problem that has been diagnosed by a physician. What is important for these people is relieving their symptoms, and the treatment looks at the underlying cause or causes of these symptoms.

My methodology

My approach is based on "precise, meticulous observation" of each individual. It seeks to discover each person's unique characteristics, offering a holistic, personalized and coherent approach. It is only by taking into account the rich complexity of each person that we can work together on an efficient preventive treatment. Truly understanding the profound richness of a person requires keeping our eyes wide open in order to be able to see and observe.

I describe the observation as "precise" because it invites us to look with a fresh approach and to appreciate a host of subtle details that we often disregard.

The observation is "meticulous" because it is systematic. By following a precise sequence of steps, we avoid hasty conclusions and learn to listen to our observations.

Each person being unique, the goal of the method is not to label everyone as a particular type, but rather to make use of typology to help us better understand ourselves. This requires a certain rigor that we must try to maintain throughout the entire morphological evaluation process.

The goal of the method is to make use of typology to help us better understand ourselves.

The book

This book will provide the answers to these two questions: "What's my type?" and "What do I have to do to look younger and feel better?" It will also provide you with the means to know yourself better and it will show you how to make the best use of your resources.

The three classical forms of medicine

Of the three oldest known forms of medicine, two are still being widely practiced but one, Greco-Roman medicine, has disappeared. It was still being taught in 17th century Europe and into the 18th century in the New World but during the second half of the 19th century it was replaced by western medicine, which is practiced in our hospitals today. Only Chinese and Indian Ayurvedic medicines are still being taught and practiced in the lands of their origins.

Their similarities

These three traditional forms of medicine originated several centuries BC. Although their diagnostic methods and therapeutic interventions are appreciably different from one another, they have several fundamental assumptions in common:

- Health is a question of balance in the body between various internal movements. These movements can be of the fluids circulating inside the body but also of emotions and thoughts. The body, emotions and thoughts all interact with one another, and disease is a signal that something has disturbed the state of equilibrium.
- A vital energy, an internal life force circulates inside the body. It is also a movement—sometimes it is several at a time—working to the benefit of the whole as well as each part. This is the source of life for each individual.

- Human beings are born with different physical, mental and emotional traits. Dominant traits are not randomly assigned; it is possible to group them into a small number of categories: three for Ayurvedic medicine, four for Greco-Roman medicine, and five for Chinese medicine. Our strengths and weaknesses are determined by the category into which we fall. The first thing you have to do is to learn how to recognize them, just as a physician would in the course of an assessment.
- The role of a physician is to help patients maintain their equilibrium (prevention) or to restore it (cure). A physician will encourage movement, remove excesses, and make up deficiencies.
- Nature will heal the sick. A physician simply facilitates nature's work. Our diet is a source of energy but we should consider it above all as a remedy available to each of us to balance excesses and deficiencies.
- Health is also a balance between the natural world and our bodies. Whatever the season, whether dry or rainy, dark or light, calm or inclement, hot or cold, we need to be aware of the effects on our bodies.

In summary, according to these traditional forms of medicine that originated over 2,000 years ago, health is a question of balance between the internal movements in the body and the external movements in our surrounding environment. We need to strive for a harmonious balance of physical exercise, nutrition, water intake, communication with our loved ones and peaceful integration into our environment. If we succeed, we might be able to live longer, better and healthier!

Some basic theory

In my anti-aging cure, I will be talking about the following concepts:

- Balance and imbalance;
- Genetic assets and genetic predisposition;
- Shape (oval, square, rectangle, circle) and color (red, green, yellow, white);
- Class of individuals who are ample (including *red ovals* and *white circles*), class of individuals who are angular (including *green squares* and *yellow rectangles*);
- Tendency.

Let me explain.

Balance and imbalance

These two terms are really at the heart of the three traditional forms of medicine to which I just referred. Here is a metaphor to help you understand them better.

People who have important or slight health problems feel as though they are sitting on a swing being bounced around in a series of disordered, uncoordinated movements. Rather than gliding back and forth in a steady, flowing arc, they lurch about in all directions, sometimes to the point of making themselves feel nauseous!

A doctor will begin by carefully observing the movements. "What's causing this person to turn this way and that?" He will pay as much attention to the swing as to the person in order to determine the cause of the problem. Perhaps the swing has become tangled. Maybe this person does not understand how to maintain the swinging motion? After having thoroughly assessed the situation, the doctor might make one or two adjustments. But even if he gives the person a push to get the swing moving freely again, he understands that it is not his role to keep it going.

A doctor can only help people by showing them how and when to propel themselves on the swing in order to achieve amplitude and rhythm in their oscillation. His role is to help someone who is sick rediscover the pleasure of the balanced motion of swinging.

Balance is
a series of
continually
occurring
adjustments,
which is
beneficial
to health.
Imbalance
is a static or
disorderly
state, which
is harmful
to health.

If you do not push yourself too high or stay stuck at the bottom, you may regain your health and equilibrium. Neither of these are static states. Both are in a constant state of self-regulating movement. We remain in good health when we are in a state of movement within an optimal zone. We get sick when we lurch about in a danger zone with no way to escape.

Balance is a series of continually occurring adjustments, which is beneficial to health. Imbalance is a static or disorderly state, which is harmful to health.

Assets and genetic predispositions

Assets are the innate gifts, or advantages, we are born with: supple and well-oxygenated skin, a metabolism that is neither too fast nor too slow, a stable nervous system, etc.

Genetic predispositions are our inherited liabilities, or disadvantages, as well as our innate advantages: skin that wrinkles easily, an over-active sympathetic nervous system, a slow lymphatic system, etc.

Hippocrates did not understand genetics, but he did isolate four major groups of advantages and disadvantages that people were born with. Today we associate these with people's genetic makeup.

You have to
learn to know
yourself better
to live better.

For individuals to live purposeful lives and to avoid sickness, Hippocrates recommended that they begin by understanding their assets and predispositions, and by being aware of them as they go about their daily lives. I could not have said it better myself. In 2,000 years, it is only the ways in which we "examine our natures" that have changed. Accordingly, in the principal sectors of health care, we have seen a refinement in procedures by which we evaluate "our natures." These new procedures are justified by the results obtained, and the measurements themselves are becoming more standardized. But the principle has not changed: you have to learn to know yourself better to live better.

Shape and color: structure and temperament

Given that the oldest forms of medicine had each classified human beings into distinct categories, I wondered how I was going to proceed.

I realized that the five elements belonging to Chinese medicine (wood, fire, earth, metal and water) and the three doshas belonging to Ayurvedic medicine (Vata, Pitta and Kapha) did not correspond to what I had observed in my practice as accurately as did the four temperaments described by Hippocrates: sanguine, bilious, nervous and lymphatic.

Consequently, I concentrated on those four categories, but quickly introduced two distinctions. First of all, rather than using the flux of the four bodily humors (blood, yellow bile, black bile and lymph) observed by Hippocrates as a starting point to define each temperament, I used the general shape of a person's body and associated a particular skin tone with each one.

That is how I established my four categories, which I call: *red oval, green square, yellow rectangle* and *white circle.*

For me, the most important feature is the skeletal structure, the body's frame. On first glance, a person's dominant shape will be clear by observing the skeletal structure.

On closer observation, looking as well as touching will help us to determine the texture and the overriding skin tone: red, green, yellow, or white. As you read on and do some of the exercises to sharpen your perception—of others and then of yourself—you will develop your own power of diagnosis.

It is important to understand here that skin colors associated with the world's main racial groups do not factor into what I have termed skin tone. An African-American could very well be classified as having the general shape of a circle and a skin tone with gray-white or pink overtones. An Asian person may blush easily and have a tone that tends towards pink, even if some people conventionally describe Asian skin as being "yellow."

I have seen so many Asians, Africans and dark-skinned people fit into the four categories of shape and color that I have stopped questioning myself! I realize that this may surprise some of my readers, but I am asking you to put your assumptions to one side

A person's dominant shape will be clear by observing the skeletal structure.

and try to look at skin differently. You will realize that there is far more to see than just the concentration of melanin!

Ample and angular

Basing myself firmly on the Hippocratic tradition, I have allowed myself to complement it with what I have observed in my professional experience.

Skin tone is an indicator of your temperamental predisposition.

These fundamental shapes—oval, square, rectangle and circle—are easier to memorize than the terms "sanguine," "bilious," "nervous," and "lymphatic." However, that is not the only reason I use them. If I talk about a *red oval,* a *green square,* a *yellow rectangle* and a *white circle,* it is because I have come to recognize the particular importance of skin tone: skin tone is an indicator of your temperamental predisposition.

These four body types can be grouped into two classes. The *green squares* and *yellow rectangles* share certain traits. I have placed them in the "angular" family. Characterized by their curves, *red ovals* and *s* make up the "ample" family.

What people of a certain type have a tendency to do

Each body type has its own distinctive characteristics. This is a simple concept that can be illustrated with a few concrete examples: *red ovals* love sweets, *green squares* hunger for savory or fatty foods, *yellow rectangles* have a passion for chocolate, and *white circles* tend to love candy.

Similarly, each body type tends towards the same choices when it comes to nutrition, exercise, skincare and interpersonal relationships. In and of themselves, these tendencies (or predispositions) are neither good nor bad. It is the possibility of doing them in excess that can pose a problem.

Distinctive traits of each shape and color

In order to determine your type, you are going to have to observe several of your physical traits. Little by little and with practice, you will develop a sure eye.

The general appearance of a body can be represented by a simple geometric shape: an oval, a rectangle, a square, or a circle. The shape of the face, shoulders, chest, torso, waist, back and thighs will help you establish the predominant geometric shape of your body or of those around you.

You can refine your observations by paying attention to facial features—the forehead, cheeks and lips—as well as to the proportions of the top part of the face relative to the middle and the lower parts.

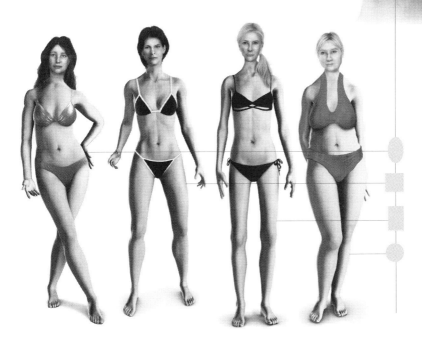

Exercises to sharpen your perception

Have you ever noticed that when you buy a new car, suddenly you see it everywhere? You never used to pay much attention to that model before, but since you bought one, you notice every one that goes by! Perception is not neutral. You perceive things to which your attention is turned. The following exercises are designed to develop your perception.

The secret to becoming an expert in the recognition of types is to practice diligently. An intellectual understanding of types is important, but it cannot take the place of careful and methodical observation. The more you observe, the faster you will become at precisely identifying the four dominant types.

Eventually it will not be a conscious effort at all to recognize the different characteristics of each type. The subtle distinctions in, for example, skin tone, muscle shape and body structure will jump out at you. You will not be able to prevent yourself from noticing them. Not only will you have acquired knowledge of typology, you will have thoroughly integrated it. That is when you will fully realize its benefits! Your friends and colleagues at work will be amazed by your "intuition," by your keen perception of them. You will develop a deeper understanding of them, as well as of yourself, each day.

It is really worth devoting time to these exercises and carefully following the instructions in order to obtain the desired results.

- Do not do more than one exercise per day.
- Do the exercises in order.
- As simple or complicated as they may seem, give them your best. The point is not necessarily to understand the exercises, but to do them.
- Relax and have confidence in yourself. If you are stressed, your internal noise will produce such a racket that you will not notice anything new. On the other hand, if you let yourself be calm and do not worry about getting it right, if you are attuned to your senses, you may be astounded by the results.
- Be flexible and accept that things may seem a little confused to begin with. This is normal when you embark on any new course of instruction.

True colors

Go and sit in a spacious restaurant, cafeteria, or any place where you can observe people without being noticed yourself. You will want to be able to see people's faces in profile as well as from the front. It will be easier for you if you concentrate on people who are sitting down. Avoid small cafés where people may feel uncomfortable at being scrutinized. A poorly lit space, such as a bar, would be difficult for this type of observation, so make sure that you choose somewhere with good lighting.

- Get comfortable. Take a few deep breaths and put all your anxieties aside.
- Look at faces without examining the details. Scan the room without trying to determine anything for the time being.
- One by one, slowly look at the skin on each face. First, identify to which class the skin of each face belongs. Does the skin fall into the yellow-green palette (angular class) or into the red–white (ample class)? If you are not sure, do not guess at the answer; simply move on to the next face. The important thing is not to be able to determine each category, but simply to learn to perceive the color palette in a face.
- Once you have had a preliminary look at each subject, refine your observation. Review each one to try to determine the skin type. Once again, it is not important if you cannot detect the dominant skin color right away. Simply move on to the next one.

Even if you end up only being able to pinpoint 10% of your subjects, you should consider the exercise a resounding success! You are honing your powers of perception, and that is what counts for the time being.

Duration: 15 minutes

The *Red Oval*

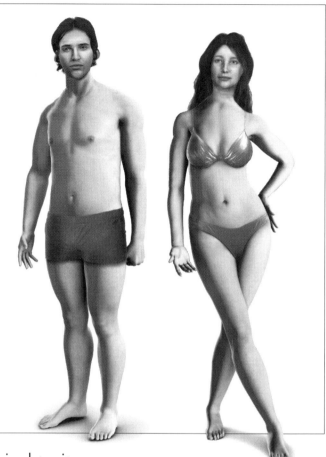

Muscles are prominent and bulky.

The face is oval-shaped.

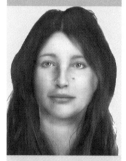

Are your bones large and solid?

Are your muscles rather large and round?

Is your waist straight?

Physical traits

Skin

First, look at the color of your skin. Skin color is the most striking feature of *red oval* types, and red is their symbolic color. *Red ovals* have more hemoglobin in their blood than other types, and this is what gives their skin this strong coloration.

If your complexion is redder than usual after a vigorous walk or exercise, your coloring becomes more pronounced if you get excited for one reason or another, or you blush easily after drinking a glass of wine or eating spicy food, then you are probably a *red oval*. But do not rush to place yourself into a category. You have several other traits to examine.

Body shape questionnaire
Red oval

By now, you will all be eager to learn what your body type is. This quick questionnaire consists of a series of yes/no questions about the physical traits that characterize each shape. There are 10 for each shape, 40 in all.

Remember that fat is not what is important. Pay attention to the bone structure and the muscles. If the hormonal system is unbalanced, it will give rise to round shapes. Knowing that, be aware of your subject's age and hormonal balance (pregnancies, menopause, endropause, etc.).

Start by reading the whole questionnaire through. When you have finished , go back to the beginning and then begin answering the questions. Score your answers as follows:
- ❖ Write 1 if your answer is yes.
- ❖ Write 0 if your answer is no.
- ❖ If you find yourself hesitating, write 0, as if the answer were no.
- ❖ If you answer yes to one element in a series, write 1.

After working through the questions in the section for each shape, add up the points for that section and compare all the totals. You will find by the end that one shape will have received more points than the others, and this will be your predominant shape.

A few words of advice:
- ❖ Do not worry: answering with a 0 does not mean you fall short in any way; it is your genetic inheritance!
- ❖ Similarly, writing 1 is not necessarily a reason to be proud!
- ❖ Do not be too hard on yourself. This is an activity to enjoy, not a final exam!
- ❖ Remember that you are measuring yourself. Never compare yourself to another person.
- ❖ If you are carrying a few extra pounds, do not worry. Fat does not count.
- ❖ Identifying what we are is a lot more difficult than identifying what we are not. So if you are unsure in any way about a question, I suggest you try a process of elimination. Just move on to the next question—or the one after that—until you find one that you know you can answer with a 1. If you are ready, let's go!

Red oval		
1	Do you look strong and solidly built?	
2	Do you have large, well-rounded muscles?	
3	Is your face oval in shape?	
4	Are your eyes, nose, or cheeks the most noticeable feature of your face? Are your cheekbones clearly visible?	
5	When you eat spicy food, drink alcohol, or stay in the sun, does your skin turn red?	
6	Are your lips naturally full?	
7	Does the strap of your bag tend to slip off your shoulder?	
8	Is your waist as wide as your shoulders?	
9	Do you sweat easily?	
10	Do your fingers and legs tend to swell during the night?	
Total out of 10:		

Bones and muscles

Are your bones large and solid?
Are your shoulders rounded? Does the strap of your bag tend to slip off your shoulder?
Are your muscles rather large and round?
Is it easy for you to blow up a balloon?
If you are a woman, do you have a nice cleavage? Voluptuous buttocks?
If you are a man, is your upper body muscular and solid?
Is your waist straight?
Do you have thickset ankles and wrists?
If you answered YES to all these questions then you are almost there.

Face

Is your face oval in shape?
Are your cheeks plump?
Are your cheekbones high and well-defined?
Overall, is your face broad?
Are your lips full and red?
Do they provide ample surface on which to apply lipstick?
Do your lips look as if they have been enhanced?
Answering YES to the majority of these questions suggests that you are mostly one type. Let's continue.

Temperature and perspiration

When you exercise, do you quickly break into a sweat? When you eat spicy food, do beads of perspiration occasionally form on your forehead? Are your hands warm? Are your feet sometimes warm in your shoes?

If you answered YES to all of these questions, you have just discovered that your type is *red oval.*

Knowing what type we are helps us to know ourselves better: more often than not, our most striking physical features go hand in hand with character traits that make up our very nature. We can get the most from our bodies and our temperaments only when we are willing to examine them and accept them for what they are. If you have discovered that your physical characteristics classify you as a *red oval,* you will be able to observe and recognize a host of character traits in yourself. Welcome them, with

We can get the most from our bodies and our temperaments only when we are willing to examine them and accept them for what they are.

all their strengths and weaknesses, and you will be able to turn them to your advantage. The anti-aging cure begins with a phase in which you will discover how to learn about yourself from the outside in.

✣

Need a massage?

*W*ho do you think could give you the best Swedish massage, assuming each was equally capable? A *red oval*, a *green square*, a *yellow rectangle*, or a *white circle?*

A person's body is not a random assemblage of parts. It is highly likely that your hands resemble your feet, the curves of your face mirror the contours of your body, and your breasts evoke the shape of your buttocks. It follows then that the hands of a *red oval* should radiate warmth. It is their natural gift. They are fleshy, powerful and sensual: perfect for a Swedish massage! The more you observe, the more you will understand how each part of the body can tell you something.

✣

Psychological traits

In general, *red ovals* need to be loved and accepted. They give what they expect to get back from others: lots of human warmth!

You are in for a real treat if you spend time with a *red oval*. They are very thoughtful and, in general, will pay attention to every little detail in creating the perfect atmosphere with just the right touches—candles, good wine, flowers and sweet nothings.

Although time spent with a *red oval* is wonderful, it is fleeting. Because, as much as they enjoy conversation, *red ovals* are fickle and always curious to know what is happening on the other side of the fence. If a neighbor has bought a new, late-model car, it will not be long before the *red oval* will want one too. Or, if another replaces his TV with a home cinema, the *red oval* will need to have one too, only with a bigger and better screen! *Red ovals* buy on impulse. Their constant cravings and insatiable desires drive the economy; they want to have the latest of everything. And if you ever need to hire top sales staff, you know that a *red oval* will be the best person to hire; they really know how to sell.

In love, they like change, particularly as regards partners. They are never happy with what they have. They are looking for fun and, like Jiminy Cricket, they live from day to day. They may

> *Red ovals* need to be loved and accepted.

be dreamers, but at least they know how to share their dreams with others. *Red ovals* like to take center stage. They know how to dress well and have a sense of decorum. They have great presence. Though they enjoy sitting at the head of the table in the place of honor, they have no desire for the responsibility that goes with it. A word of advice, then: do not talk to *red ovals* about their responsibilities. They much prefer that things remain simple and uncomplicated.

Their keen powers of observation, appreciation for beauty and desire to be noticed would make them acclaimed designers, excellent architects, or famous chefs.

They understand how to present food on a plate, how to place the plate on a table and how to arrange the table in a resplendent room. They can easily promote their cause and convincingly defend their point of view.

Oh! If only the *red oval* could have your house! *Red ovals* might lust after your wine cellar, grand piano, leather sofa, fur coat, jewelry, or your Hermès purse or suitcase. They are never satisfied with what they have and always yearn for what they do not have.

In an elevator, they will always be able to recognize your perfume. Distinguishing Chanel No. 5 from Calvin Klein's Obsession is child's play for them! If wine arouses their interest, you can bet they will be able to tell a Clos de Vougeot Burgundy from a Saint-Émilion Bordeaux—merely by smelling its aroma! They know all the finest vintages and, keen to impress, they may even teach you about wine tasting.

Connoisseurs of life, self-absorbed, they feed off good food as much as lavish compliments. And because of this, they can be easily influenced. However, they fly off the handle easily. Do not ever dare ask them, "Have you put on a few pounds?" They will take it very badly, even if it is true, and may be stirred into a rage, instantly turning them a bright shade of red!

Moreover, you should never contradict a *red oval* or rub them the wrong way! Always be diplomatic with them. If by chance you should happen to say the wrong thing, however, do not worry: an hour later, they will have forgotten all about it! Yet no matter what you say to them, they will never let it interfere with their digestion nor their sleep. For them, tomorrow is another day.

Assets and genetic predispositions

You realize now that *red ovals* have many assets up their sleeves.

As far as relationships go, they know how to make themselves indispensable and how to be everywhere at once so as not to miss anything. They are terrific listeners. They know how to get anything they need in just the right manner; they do not manipulate people, but they understand how to put them at ease to gain their confidence. Indeed, people will feel comfortable telling a *red oval* things they would not repeat to anyone else. *Red ovals* have entire networks of acquaintances and keep in touch with everyone.

They will often commit sins of excess, but are the first to put themselves back on the straight and narrow when counseled. When they realize that the good advice they are being given will only help them, they appreciate and are even grateful for it. Fashion-conscious and sensitive to what is acceptable and what is not, *red ovals* would happily go on a diet or follow a regimen to improve their figure.

Beautiful skin

Red ovals are blessed with a major genetic asset. They have beautiful skin, well-oxygenated and firm, which hardly wrinkles. If they burn themselves anywhere on the body, their skin will scar rapidly. Theirs is the skin that scars the most beautifully! They will not wrinkle with age, though they may develop unflattering red blotches. They are prime candidates for all types of rosacea.

Red ovals are blessed with a major genetic asset. They have beautiful skin that hardly wrinkles.

If you have ever heard a friend say, "My mother didn't use any creams and never got a single wrinkle. I don't believe in creams!" you can assure your friend that she inherited a wonderful gift from her mother: a skin that will stand the test of time, the skin of a *red oval!*

Sales persons for skin and beauty products whose own skin demonstrates the beneficial effects of their products are, more often than not, *red ovals.* They do not need these products for themselves, as they already naturally possess clear and beautiful skin.

Nevertheless, one out of every two clients in beauty salons and spas is a *red oval.* Why is this? Well, for two excellent reasons: first, *red ovals* care about their appearance, and second, they are easily influenced. They are not there for the relaxation; they want to look good!

❖

Sara, or when to start thinking about anti-aging

Sometimes people ask me, "At what age should one begin to think about anti-aging? 25 years old, 30, 40, 50? What do you think?"

I like to respond to that by talking about someone very dear to me—my daughter Sara. Sara, at 3, was blessed with her father's *red oval* beautiful skin, invigorated and smooth, with good blood circulation and a splendid color. I knew then that wrinkles would never take hold of her face. A gift, courtesy of her genes!

Even so, some areas of redness were visible on her face. Upon closer observation, it looked as though she would be a prime candidate for rosacea. If heredity works to our advantage in some areas, it can also predispose us to certain problems in others.

My professional bias has resulted in a preoccupation with some of these issues, which borders on the obsessive. Still a toddler, Sara neither knew how to read nor count. Yet her mother was already worried about preserving her youth! This might seem absurd.

Well, not entirely. Anti-aging is based on knowledge of oneself. The root of this self-knowledge is meticulous observation and an understanding of body types. As I see it, anti-aging is not an obsession with eternal youth, but simply a sound and intelligent way to live in good health and age gracefully; we can prevent the passage of time from leaving its mark on us due to self-neglect.

Sara is a beautiful little girl. Knowing her genetic heritage, I take simple preventive measures to ensure her overall well-being. I know that her skin is sensitive to the sun, so I protect her from harmful UVA and UVB rays. *Red ovals* are more sensitive and are, therefore, predisposed to skin cancer, which might prove fatal to them. I avoid giving her hot baths, as they might accentuate the red blotches on her skin over time.

An understanding of body types is as important for children as it is for adults. If your young daughter is clearly a *white circle*, you might want to consider taking some preventive measures now. If you do not, when she reaches adolescence with all its hormonal changes, she might well turn into a little round ball of lymph! While this evidently will not change her worth as a human being, it will certainly affect her self-image. To ensure her future wellbeing, you can take one or two simple measures now: make sure her diet is adapted to her needs and encourage her to get the right type of exercise.

❖

Predispositions

The predominant genetic disposition of *red ovals*, their principal physical weakness, is their vascular and circulatory imbalance. Predisposed to high blood pressure, *red ovals* should beware of their tendency to over-eating and over-drinking. They love to taste everything, but have to realize that the downside is a round shape and being overweight. The redness on their skin is a consequence of high blood pressure.

They have a tendency towards:

- Allergies
- Angina
- Arrhythmia
- Asthma
- Blood clots (strokes, thrombosis, pulmonary embolism)
- Diabetes
- Edema
- Fibromyalgia
- Gout
- High blood pressure
- High cholesterol (high levels of low-density lipoprotein, or LDL)
- Inflammatory arthritis
- Kidney disease
- Palpitations
- Chubbiness
- Rosacea
- Soft (hydric) cellulite
- Thyroid gland imbalance
- Venous insufficiency
- Weak immune system

Because a *red oval's* skin has a thin epidermal layer and a dermis full of blood vessels, it is perfectly oxygenated. You might see some red blotches on a *red oval's* face, which may be a precursor to rosacea that could worsen with time. Female *red ovals* may develop cellulite, but this is easily treatable.

Even if a *red oval's* good humor, joie de vivre and happy-go-lucky attitude allow them to forget all their predispositions towards heart disease and red blotches, they are susceptible to still another series of health problems.

If they injure themselves, they will avoid looking at the wound because, in general, they cannot stand the sight of blood. They would rather have someone else look after them and will generally follow instructions carefully on how to take care of themselves following an injury.

Everything is a question of degree. A *red oval* is neither better nor worse than anyone else. They simply have to understand their essential natures and what they have to work with. Their dilemma is the same as everybody else's: finding the right balance.

But nature is even-handed: for each type, advantages compensate for disadvantages. A *red oval* is susceptible to redness, but at the same time has beautiful firm and well-oxygenated skin. It is up to you to discover your own strengths and weaknesses. This book is precisely designed to help you understand how your nature works to your advantage as well as to your disadvantage.

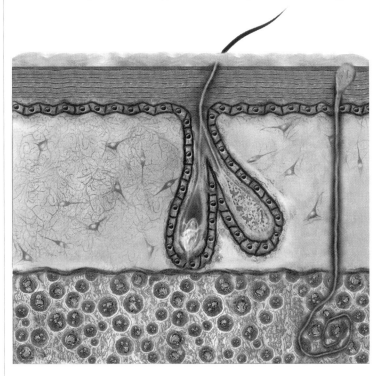

Thin epidermis, thick dermis, well-vascularized.

The *Green Square*

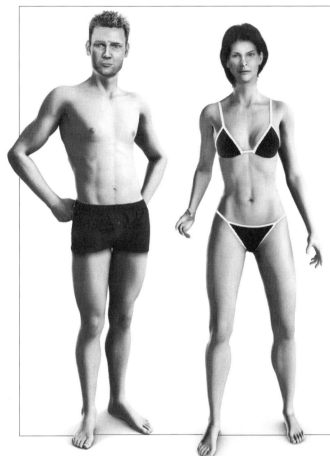

Shape of general body structure is a square or a triangle.

The three zones of the face are equally proportioned

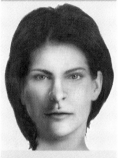

Overall, would you say your body is well-proportioned?

Are your muscles of medium size and well-balanced?

Is your jawline square?

Physical traits

The most striking traits in a *green square* are, of course, the well-proportioned body and broad shoulders that taper to a slender waist. Their next most compelling characteristic is the balance evident in the perfect proportions between all the parts of the body. They possess what is considered the ideal shape: square shoulders, slender and well-defined waist (even when they gain weight) and long, tapered legs.

Green squares are the typical embodiment of beauty as we perceive it today:

Prominent, well-defined traits;
Slightly rounded forehead;
Shapely and equally proportioned lips;
Slim waist;

Perfect legs: not too long nor too thin;

Medium bone structure, perfectly proportioned;

In women, breasts are separated and bones in the upper chest are slightly discernible;

In men, bones in the upper chest are also slightly discernible;

Muscles are well-formed and sculpted. *Green squares* do not seem to need to go to the gym to look athletic! But if they did work out, their already handsome physiques would rapidly develop even further.

Green squares are often "full of bile," especially when they are tired or overworked. Bile is black and through the skin appears green. Indeed, their olive-green coloring is a result of this condition.

Perspiration and temperature

Another characteristic trait of a *green square* is the tendency towards cold hands, feet and sometimes the tip of their nose when stressed or fatigued. They live off their adrenalin: their blood flows to the heart and the muscles to ensure their mobility, and the blood vessels in their extremities constrict, resulting in a drop in skin temperature.

In front of a microphone or an audience, where they may suddenly develop stage fright, *green squares* may get sweaty hands. But the rest of their body will be dry. When they take a sauna, *green squares* notice that they sweat less than others. Likewise, if they have a hot body wrap in a spa, they will feel that the treatment is not working. They eliminate very little by way of the skin and compensate by putting great demands on their internal organs, notably the liver and kidneys.

Psychological traits

Green squares like to be in control. They want the last word. They know it all—or at least pretend to. They are sure of themselves and are extroverted, and they express their opinions, even when not invited to. They will unabashedly pour their hearts out in front of people, in contrast to *red ovals* who are content brooding quietly to themselves.

Professionally ambitious, they will embark on several projects at a time. They are highly demanding of themselves and even more so of others.

Body shape questionnaire
Green square

By now, you will all be eager to learn what your body type is. This quick questionnaire consists of a series of yes/no questions about the physical traits that characterize each shape. There are 10 for each shape, 40 in all.

Remember that fat is not what is important. Pay attention to the bone structure and the muscles. If the hormonal system is unbalanced, it will give rise to round shapes. Knowing that, be aware of your subject's age and hormonal balance (pregnancies, menopause, endropause, etc.).

Start by reading the whole questionnaire through. When you have finished , go back to the beginning and then begin answering the questions. Score your answers as follows:
- ❖ Write 1 if your answer is yes.
- ❖ Write 0 if your answer is no.
- ❖ If you find yourself hesitating, write 0, as if the answer were no.
- ❖ If you answer yes to one element in a series, write 1.

After working through the questions in the section for each shape, add up the points for that section and compare all the totals. You will find by the end that one shape will have received more points than the others, and this will be your predominant shape.

A few words of advice:

- ❖ Do not worry: answering with a 0 does not mean you fall short in any way; it is your genetic inheritance!
- ❖ Similarly, writing 1 is not necessarily a reason to be proud!
- ❖ Do not be too hard on yourself. This is an activity to enjoy, not a final exam!
- ❖ Remember that you are measuring yourself. Never compare yourself to another person.
- ❖ If you are carrying a few extra pounds, do not worry. Fat does not count.
- ❖ Identifying what we are is a lot more difficult than identifying what we are not. So if you are unsure in any way about a question, I suggest you try a process of elimination. Just move on to the next question—or the one after that—until you find one that you know you can answer with a 1. If you are ready, let's go!

Green square	
1.	Overall, would you say that you have a well-proportioned body?	
2.	Do you have well-proportioned, average-sized and well-shaped muscles?	
3.	If you place your chin on the table, does it feel square-shaped?	
4.	Are your lips of average size?	
5.	Do you have an olive skin tone?	
6.	Are your shoulders wider than your waist?	
7.	Do you have a slender waist?	
8.	Do your hands and feet often feel cold for no apparent reason?	
9.	Are your nasal labial folds (beginning at the wings of the nose extending down to your chin) deep and visible?	
10.	If you place a hand on the top of your chest, can you easily feel your bones?	
Total out of 10:	

Green squares are extremely skeptical and need solid proof before being convinced of anything. But once they believe in something, they will promote their views with ardor. *Green squares* often get too caught up in the details, which tends to exasperate those around them.

Moreover, they tend to become consumed by any endeavor they undertake: they do not tire and certainly are not concerned that others might. *Green squares* push ahead relentlessly and, if someone falls behind, they have the strength to pick them up and pull them along. Constantly active, they would rather skip a meal than fall behind in their work.

At home, a woman who is a *green square* will be as likely to stay in pajamas as to keep her hair in rollers all day, and a man will wear sweatpants and not worry about his unkempt hair. Neither one will give it a second thought as they keep themselves busy all day. Their poorly groomed appearance does not worry them in the least because they know that it is their energy and vigor that people admire most in them. Being sloppy around the house is, for them, a form of relaxation, the only one they will permit themselves. On the other hand, if they go out with friends, you can be sure that, of the entire group, they will be the ones wearing the most exclusive items.

Green squares do not want to disappoint. Mostly, they do not want to disappoint themselves! In fact, they are not really all that concerned about other people's opinions (unless they pertain to themselves or their family). They set the bar very high for themselves and are extremely guarded about admitting their weaknesses to others. They will either keep them to themselves, or confide only in those of whose support they can be assured. Above all, they want to project an air of strength and assurance. Yet they are still able to cry alone in their room or in front of those close to them. They have big hearts, but do not like to parade them in public.

There is always a clear motive to what *green squares* do. Any undertaking has to reap a benefit. It could be financial in nature, the admiration to be gained from others, or simply the personal satisfaction at having accomplished something. A *green square* does not do something to be fashionable. In contrast to *red ovals,* who need to be "in," *green squares* could not care less. If what they do is based on their convictions and it achieves their desired objective, that is all that matters. A *red oval* needs to conform and a *green square* desires to be unique.

Red ovals acquire things to show off the fact that they have the financial means to do so. *Green squares,* on the other hand, buy exclusive items for their own sake—and never pay full price! They are formidable negotiators and will haggle over the price with a seller, down to the last nickel, for a better deal. *Green squares* have an eye for bargains and can often be found at sales and auctions. The day after Christmas, like *red ovals,* they turn into frenzied shoppers, but not for the same reasons. *Red ovals* simply want to get what they have seen at their friends' houses, whereas green squares are looking to acquire those one-of-a-kind items at a bargain!

Green squares cannot stop thinking ahead and are plagued by anxieties and a multitude of preoccupations. They plan, they anticipate constantly and are always imagining the worst. They have difficulty relaxing. And on the rare occasions when they do, by the pool for example, they do not stop thinking about work or their children. They are simply unable to live from day to day, unlike the thoroughly carefree *red ovals.*

Guilt is a perpetual state of being for them: they go on vacation, they go on a guilt trip; they work hard, they feel guilty. Whatever they do, guilt is part of the package.

Green squares will be able to tell you all about the relaxation techniques found in yoga or meditation, but generally will never sign up for a class themselves. But if someone else were finally able to convince them to go, or if for some other reason they had to participate in a class, they would, indeed, apply themselves completely and be very good students.

Holiday celebrations or a parent or friend's birthday would be good reasons for a *green square* to allow themselves to take a break. If they offer someone a gift, it has to be original and unique so that the person receiving them is completely thrilled and delighted. *Green squares* have to be in control, even when they are giving. That being said, do not count on receiving anything from them; their decisions verge on the extreme, and they may simply decide not to give a gift at all.

When disgruntled, a *green square* will not hesitate to let you know. If they have a bad experience, such as in a restaurant, they will make sure everyone around them is aware of it and may even exaggerate the initial cause of their irritation. However, they are loyal and enjoy what is familiar and may eventually return to this same restaurant. Owners should be keenly aware of their *green*

Green squares cannot stop thinking ahead and are plagued by anxieties and a multitude of preoccupations.

⁘

Learn to unwind!

I was having dinner in a restaurant with one of the people in charge of a large American company, along with one of his associates. I did not know either of them, but had once met their boss. While waiting in the lobby to be seated, we began to discuss business. During the course of the conversation, the associate confided in me, "At the office, the boss is a bit cold. It is hard to know what he's thinking." I told her that I had met him only once, had shaken his hand, and had arrived at the conclusion that he fit into the category of green square.

She wanted to know what I meant. I went on to explain that I was writing a book on the four main body types people fall into and on the complete anti-aging cure for each of them, according to their body type.

Her colleague, who was following the conversation, then asked, "And me, what type am I?" I took some time to examine him and said, "Your type is predominantly green square, with a little yellow rectangle." He asked me what that meant. I explained that he had a tendency towards premature aging, adding that what was causing him to age at that moment was the accumulation of too many projects going on at the same time. If he wanted to get involved in the anti-aging cure, he would have to begin by learning how to relax.

He was surprised by this answer. "Learn to relax?" He turned to his colleague and asked her if he seemed tense. She replied that she found him anxious. I continued, saying that his metabolism was very fast. I told him that there was a correlation between the fact that he could think and act quickly and that he burned calories just as fast. His nervous system was having an impact on his hormonal system, which, in turn, was having an impact on his metabolism.

I added that he would probably soon be experiencing problems with his colon. His skin was poorly oxygenated and he would develop wrinkles from his various facial expressions. What would help him, I explained, was not anti-wrinkle cream, but taking a break, yoga, music—in short, deep and profound relaxation.

He then observed, "I've never met anyone who could tell me as much about myself in such a short space of time as you have. I'm going to buy your book!" Once seated at our table, we resumed our business conversation, but he frequently referred back to the four body types and the anti-aging cure that was appropriate to him.

⁘

square clients: these are the ones to look after with kid gloves because they will ultimately be the restaurant's best ambassadors if they are satisfied with the food or the service. Moreover, they will naturally let it be known that they enjoy being pampered with special treats!

Green squares hate to waste time. Never be late for a meeting with a *green square;* you will never hear the end of it. Nevertheless, *green squares* will think nothing of being late themselves, if it serves their purpose.

Assets and genetic predispositions

Psychological assets

Green squares are visionaries who take action. They are entrepreneurs and enjoy competition and challenge. They are autonomous and well-organized, and they know how to delegate to get everybody working. If you are looking for a manager for an important project, do not hesitate to select a *green square.* They will handle it as well as, if not better, than you. They will display leadership. If tensions and difficulties arise, they will confront them and find solutions to problems in all areas. Their perfectionist tendencies make them exceptional human beings. They might be moody, but they get things done.

Physical assets

Green squares are well-proportioned and attractive. Though they may not do any particular exercise, most *green squares* look athletic and have well-defined physiques. To see them, you would say they have everything going for them.

Genetic predispositions

They are used to being leaders, and consider work before their health. *Green squares* push themselves to the limit without making sure to care for their inherent weaknesses.

Nevertheless, just as for the others, they have many. Take backache, for example. You do not need to be a massage therapist to know that *green squares* are bound to their work and only consult a therapist when it is almost too late! They wait until they are well and truly in the grip of excruciating lower back pain before they will go and get help. Even when they are doubled over, they are still thinking about falling behind schedule in their work.

They want relief and they want it now! They are not really listening to the messages their body is sending them. Pain is a waste of time to them. In fact, *green squares* really hate to have to stop working—unless, of course, they can somehow turn it to their advantage!

The skin of a *green square* has a thick epidermis and a thin dermis with poor circulation. This is a genetic predisposition that could lead to many kinds of skin problems:

- Wrinkles from facial expressions. These form rapidly as the epidermis and dermis become detached from one another;
- Skin discoloration. These are not freckles or birthmarks, but brown marks that appear on the face, called hyperpigmentation. An alternate name for this disorder is melasma. Though unattractive, melasma is not dangerous;
- Stretch marks following pregnancy;
- Milia. These are tiny white bumps made of small masses of hard fat trapped under the surface of the skin. They can get bigger with time. They may be removed by a doctor but have patience; they will disappear on their own;

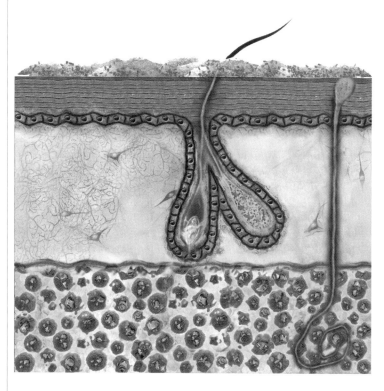

Thick epidermis, thin dermis, poorly vascularized.

- Cellulite. The cellulite on a *green square* is compact, hard and fibrous. It appears as dimples on the legs, stomach, arms and thighs. In women, this type of cellulite is particularly unattractive and, therefore, the least tolerated;
- Scarring. Scar tissue on their skin does not heal very well. If they have to undergo surgery, the skin should be well prepared in advance. Following surgery, it is recommended to supplement the natural healing process;
- Nervous system. If their nervous systems are taxed too highly from stress, they can become imbalanced, possibly resulting in the development of eczema, psoriasis, or cystic acne. The skin could become excessively oily or, conversely, excessively dry;
- Keloids. *Green squares* are prone to developing keloids (fibrous, bumpy scar tissue).

In summary, *green squares* have a tendency towards:

- Adrenal insufficiency
- Alzheimer's disease
- Anemia
- Anxiety
- Arteriosclerosis
- Attention-deficit disorder (ADD)
- Cancer
- Carpal tunnel syndrome
- Fibrosis
- Fibrous cellulite
- Fibrous tumors
- Hepatitis
- Hypoglycemia
- Insomnia
- Irritable bowel syndrome (IBS)
- Keloids
- Low blood pressure
- Milia (tiny whiteheads)
- Multiple sclerosis
- Osteoarthritis
- Osteoporosis
- Psoriasis
- Stretch marks

The last genetic trait that *green squares* need to be keenly aware of is their predisposition towards bad cholesterol. *Green squares* tend to develop atherosclerosis, or hardening of the arteries. The arteries gradually become clogged by a buildup of atheroma, or fatty deposits, inside the walls. Eventually, the arteries grow narrower, and the flow of blood is affected. A small clot can become blocked in the artery, and, if this is a coronary artery, this can lead to a heart attack.

When *green squares* do not manage to control their weaknesses, the result may be that stress takes over, and they end up permanently functioning on adrenaline, which is exhausting to the body. They do everything to hasten the aging process.

They can also suffer from a number of serious ailments: Crohn's disease (a disease of the colon), osteoporosis and Alzheimer's disease. The blessings of their genetic advantages just are not strong enough to counterbalance their disadvantages. Indeed, it is often the over reliance on and abuse of their strengths that lead to their health problems.

Tumors and fibrosis. The pressure and stress common to *green squares* can be risk factors for the development of cancer.

The danger they face is that they may become overanxious and develop insomnia. They can go so far as to have suicidal

❖

Stretch marks and my professional preoccupation!

uring my first pregnancy, knowing my body type, I gave myself three strict instructions: cream, cream, cream, then added a further three: oil, oil, oil! I possess some very pronounced green square traits, and I understood that I would have to slather on huge amounts of rejuvenating and regenerating creams and oils daily if I were to avoid stretch marks. The epidermis of a green square is thicker, more detached from the dermis and less nourished by blood vessels; any weight gain or sudden loss of weight could easily produce stretch marks.

I really had no excuse for ignorance, and I certainly had at my disposal all the creams that I could possibly need, so I told myself that this, indeed, was the moment to practice what I preached! It might surprise you to learn that a skin-care professional needed a little motivation in order to treat herself with a few skin-care basics, but remember, this skin-care professional is also—a green square! It is in the nature of green squares to be less concerned than other types about taking care of themselves.

Accordingly, every morning, without exception and with much determination (another green square tendency), I smeared my tummy with creams and oils. I used gallons of the stuff! I basted myself like a turkey!

After my first child, Adam, was born—a beautiful baby weighing 10.5 pounds—there was not a single stretch mark to be seen on my tummy. Read between the lines: not one on my tummy!

Well, you can be sure that now I explain clearly to green squares—whose natural tendency is to neglect their skin—that they have to take care of the skin on their entire bodies during pregnancy!

❖

tendencies and to develop psychosomatic pain. This is related to their inability to unwind and enjoy life, because of the numerous projects they undertake at once with all the conflicts that that can produce.

When imbalanced, *green squares* can exhibit traits that do them a great disservice. They can become so competitive that they are a danger to themselves and others. They can fight fiercely against an adversary, putting aside all ethical considerations for the sheer thrill of winning. They do not like to lose. They can destroy a colleague who had the misfortune to express a contrary opinion. Their behavior can become abusive, extreme and manipulative.

Exercise to sharpen your perception

Exercise 2.

Moving colors

Find a spot close to the exit of a subway, in a shopping mall, or on a busy sidewalk. Try to be unobtrusive so that people will not feel uncomfortable at being observed.

❖ Relax. Take a few deep breaths and leave all your other thoughts aside. The rhythm of this exercise is more rapid than the previous one, but you should not let this make you tense. The more tense you are, the less attuned you will be to your senses.

❖ Look at faces without scrutinizing the details. You will only have a few seconds to observe the skin. As people go by, let yourself linger on one or two faces. Does the skin fall into the color palette of the angular class of individuals or into the color palette of the ample class of individuals? If the answer comes to you quickly, so much the better. If not, simply move on to the next one.

Just as in the preceding exercise, the number of identified faces is not a measure of success. If you are only able to categorize a few people with certainty, you have been successful.

Duration: 5 minutes

The *Yellow Rectangle*

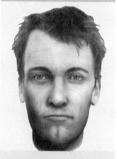

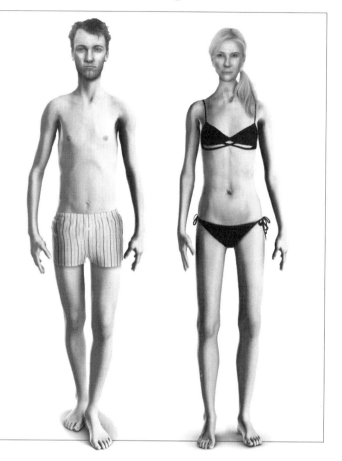

Physical traits

Bones and muscles

Seen from a distance, people who belong to the *yellow rectangle* category look tall and slender, even gangly and skeletal.

Their shoulders are narrow and often very straight. Their bones are quite visible. In relation to the rest of their body, their torso and arms are proportionately long and skinny. Women are flat-chested and you can see their ribs, especially when you observe them breathing or lying down (unless they have had breast implants).

Their waists are thin and narrow. The pelvic bones are very noticeable. Dancers are often *yellow rectangles*. Their frames are

Body shape questionnaire
Yellow rectangle

By now, you will all be eager to learn what your body type is. This quick questionnaire consists of a series of yes/no questions about the physical traits that characterize each shape. There are 10 for each shape, 40 in all.

Remember that fat is not what is important. Pay attention to the bone structure and the muscles. If the hormonal system is unbalanced, it will give rise to round shapes. Knowing that, be aware of your subject's age and hormonal balance (pregnancies, menopause, endropause, etc.).

Start by reading the whole questionnaire through. When you have finished , go back to the beginning and then begin answering the questions. Score your answers as follows:
- ❖ Write 1 if your answer is yes.
- ❖ Write 0 if your answer is no.
- ❖ If you find yourself hesitating, write 0, as if the answer were no.
- ❖ If you answer yes to one element in a series, write 1.

After working through the questions in the section for each shape, add up the points for that section and compare all the totals. You will find by the end that one shape will have received more points than the others, and this will be your predominant shape.

A few words of advice:
- ❖ Do not worry: answering with a 0 does not mean you fall short in any way; it is your genetic inheritance!
- ❖ Similarly, writing 1 is not necessarily a reason to be proud!
- ❖ Do not be too hard on yourself. This is an activity to enjoy, not a final exam!
- ❖ Remember that you are measuring yourself. Never compare yourself to another person.
- ❖ If you are carrying a few extra pounds, do not worry. Fat does not count.
- ❖ Identifying what we are is a lot more difficult than identifying what we are not. So if you are unsure in any way about a question, I suggest you try a process of elimination. Just move on to the next question—or the one after that—until you find one that you know you can answer with a 1. If you are ready, let's go!

Yellow rectangle	
1	Bones. Are they fine and delicate?	
2	Are your muscles long and streamlined and not well-defined?	
3	Do you rarely blush? Is your skin pale?	
4	Would you say there is a yellowish tone to your skin?	
5	Looking at your face, is your forehead the most noticeable feature, is your chin pointed?	
6	Are your lips narrow?	
7	Do you think you have narrow, straight shoulders?	
8	Is the top part of your body slender and slim?	
9	Do you have a dancer's legs (long and slim)?	
10	Do you always feel cold?	
Total out of 10:	

light and their bones can be discerned under the skin. However, they differ from *green squares* in two respects:

- The muscles of a *yellow rectangle* are long and lean. They can be strong, but they take up very little bulk;
- The bones of a *yellow rectangle* are light and frail.

Face

Their faces are predominantly rectangular. Sometimes they can be in the shape of a triangle. The most prominent feature is the forehead. Their lips are thin, and the corners of their mouths are often turned down as though they were unhappy!

Skin

Poorly oxygenated and in most cases inadequately cared for, their skin looks pallid and anemic. Their complexion looks like that of yellow parchment. Even in a state of high emotion, the skin of a *yellow rectangle* will not flush. The epidermis is thick, and the dermis is very thin—even more so than that of a *green square*. It has few blood vessels nourishing it. It contains few fibroblasts, produces little collagen and, as a result, lacks elasticity and resilience. If they burn themselves anywhere on the body, *yellow rectangles* will scar, and the scar will not heal well and will remain visible.

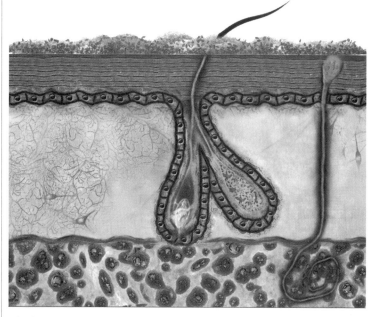

Thick epidermis, very thin dermis, poorly vascularized, contains few fibroblasts.

Nervous system and metabolism

Yellow rectangles have rapid nervous systems that work very hard. It is both their major strength and their greatest weakness.

They can eat constantly, but never get fat because they burn all their calories. If *white circles* were to eat as much, they would certainly become obese!

Temperature and perspiration

Yellow rectangles are always cold and always worry about getting cold. If they have to speak in public, their hands get clammy due to the demands made on their nervous systems. They rarely sweat, even when they exercise, with two exceptions: occasionally, their feet will sweat in their shoes and / or will often break out in a cold sweat at night. These sweats are frequently related to nightmares and, hence, the feverish quality of their cerebral activity.

Psychological traits

Yellow rectangles are introverts. They enjoy routine and follow regular schedules that they have established themselves. They like to share their opinions, but not in front of just anybody. They appreciate good conversation with friends and have no interest in impressing ignoramuses who do not belong to their inner circle.

They dread public speaking and prefer to talk to people on a one-to-one basis. Where they shine is in front of a select group of friends. It takes a long time to earn their trust, but once you do, it will be forever.

Yellow rectangles love to go for walks in the woods. They are independent and often single. As much as they cherish and are loyal to their friends, they also enjoy being alone. Furthermore, although they do not express their feelings verbally, they are very emotional and generally do not forget someone's birthday. They are attentive to others, understand their needs well and take great pleasure in satisfying their desires.

Great lovers and staunch defenders of nature, they are eminently respectful of the environment and abhor cruelty to animals. They recycle with zeal and carry their groceries in paper bags. They are often macrobiotics, vegetarians, or even vegans. They seem to be mostly drawn to being vegans—those who avoid all animal products, including eggs and dairy products, eating only fruits and vegetables. Some vegans will restrict their diets to raw

They can eat constantly, but never get fat because they burn all their calories.

Yellow rectangles are introverts. They enjoy routine.

foods and eliminate all processed foods. In general, *yellow rectangles* will buy their foods in health food stores or in the organic sections of their supermarkets.

Yellow rectangles are dependable and self-controlled. They enjoy playing with children, willingly letting down their guard, relaxing and joining in the simplest of games.

They like sports and discipline.

When they give of their time or money, they ask for nothing in return. Although they may at times appear envious, they are really quite content with what they have.

Yellow rectangles do not worry about their appearance. They believe that beauty establishments are not for them. Nevertheless, if they receive a gift certificate for a beauty treatment or a massage, their curiosity will be piqued, and they will take the opportunity to ask a slew of questions! Before buying anything, they always want more information about the product. The problem is that answers to their questions only breed more questions! Perpetually anxious, *yellow rectangles* are intent on gathering information about anything and everything. "Are you sure this product has not been tested on animals?" "Will this shot hurt?" The apprehension that lurks behind their quest for knowledge is sometimes hard to hide. They dislike gadgets and new technology, yet sometimes the sheer number of questions they direct at a salesperson will make them look like experts on the subject!

They talk quickly, hardly leaving themselves time to catch their breath. On occasion, they will even talk in their sleep! Even so, they often give the impression of being calm and self-possessed. On the inside, though, a *yellow rectangle's* metabolism is working frantically. Their thoughts flow rapidly and uninterruptedly, but their anxiety is never far behind.

The world of knowledge or abstract thinking fascinates them. They always want to learn more. *Yellow rectangles* never waste time reading novels; they read to become informed and instructed, or to confirm or reinforce a currently held belief or lifestyle choice. They appreciate the world of theory and experimental research. They feel confident when everything is based on fact and measurable. They love to explain what they know—even if the explanations can sometimes be a bit lengthy for those listening!

It is not uncommon, then, to find *yellow rectangles* teaching or doing research. They are cerebral, but they can be inflexible. They value coherent systems of explanation based on reason. Often exceptionally erudite in their domain, they are not always able to transmit their knowledge in lay terms. Many are specialists in a field of activity and are not interested in broadening their scope. As artists, musicians, or writers, they are highly inventive and give full rein to their creativity with great intensity.

❖

Buy like a *yellow rectangle*, dress like a *red oval*

I travel frequently, so I always make sure to call and talk to my children every day, sometimes even several times a day! I remember, in particular, the time that my son Samy answered the phone. I had just finished saying, "Hello...," when he answered, "Fine!" I answered, "Samy, I haven't asked you how you are yet; I only got as far as saying hello!" He continued, "Hi, Mom, I'm fine, I've done my homework, I've had my supper, and now I'm going to play with my friends." From the start of the conversation, he knew what would follow. Samy, a predominant *yellow rectangle*, is as fast as this body type gets. Nothing computes slowly in his head. Typical!

Yellow rectangles have exceptional mental abilities. Things that may be confusing for other types can be easily processed by a *yellow rectangle*. But do not be fooled! Their minds are, indeed, quick and sharp, but their actions do not flow spontaneously from their thoughts. In fact, many *yellow rectangles* bring new meaning to the adage "look before you leap." They will mull something over and over, driving themselves crazy in the process, but then will invariably fail to take any action!

While visiting New York with my family, Samy, my *yellow rectangle* son, waited until the very last day to do his shopping because he wanted to make sure he had carefully considered his choices. My son Adam, on the other hand, leagues away from being a *yellow rectangle*, arrived in New York with his shopping list at the ready. Like his father, with whom he shares some striking *red oval* traits, his penchant was for the trendy and fashionable. I have long given up ironing shirts for my husband, Amir. Pragmatic *green square* that I am, I never seem to be able to iron them with the finesse and attention to detail required by his *red oval* elegance. He irons them himself now, happy in the knowledge that they are being done to his satisfaction.

❖

Yellow rectangles are attracted to professions that require strict adherence to rules.

Yellow rectangles are also attracted to professions that require strict adherence to rules. They can often be found in fields in which the professional mindset is informed by anxiety, insecurity, or uncertainty: government worker, border guard, soldier, etc. They do not live in the present, but in the future: they analyze everything, elaborating all manner of hypotheses and scenarios. If they work in information technology, they are experts in 3D computer modeling or any branch that requires concentrated cerebral activity.

They can be counted among some of the greatest artists. Their flair for language makes them writers, poets and teachers, their talent for innovation in three-dimensional form produces sculptors, and their eye for color and texture encourages them to become painters. They are also great musicians.

As they are generally in constant fear of losing their jobs, they sometimes donate their time to make themselves indispensable. They gripe about those who are better off than they are. They have no marketing skills and have no wish to acquire any. Products hold less importance for them than the ideas that helped conceive them. They do not trust salespeople and are skeptical of what a seller will tell them.

They save their money and have no debts. They regularly pay off the exact amount owing on their credit cards. When they purchase something, it is not to enjoy their possessions nor to solicit envy from others, but simply to acquire what they need.

Nonetheless, the *yellow rectangle* is certainly capable of being opportunistic. While *green squares* will be concerned with their own interests first, and while *red ovals* will seize an opportunity if it seems like a good way to raise their standing in society, *yellow rectangles* will only look to gain something from those who are more knowledgeable than themselves. For example, they may seek the opinion of an expert to improve upon certain findings of their own. Their tendency will be to try to extract information from such a person, to put it to their own use. This is an example of the *yellow rectangle's* two underlying preoccupations: to seek out those who know and to be constantly learning new things.

They are perfectly happy to have several things on the burner at once. However, paradoxically, they may feel overwhelmed by the variety of tasks requested of them. They are obsessed by the idea that they cannot have a moment's rest, which leads them to swing between being alternately hypervigilant and negligent. They demand so much of their intellects that sometimes things escape them. Their attention is focused exclusively on the task at hand, but having so many things going on at once makes it seem as if they never finish anything! In fact, they do get through things, but they need to understand that the most effective way for them to accomplish anything is to not accept too many tasks at once. Understand, of course, that this tendency of theirs to bite off more than they can chew is linked to the fact that they cannot say no!

Assets and genetic predispositions

Yellow rectangles have two major assets: their exceptional intellectual abilities and their rapid metabolism. They possess all the aptitudes needed to learn, understand and assimilate; however, they may not be able to demonstrate everything that they have learned. On the other hand, they can eat absolutely anything they want without gaining any weight.

Nonetheless, they need to pay attention to four genetic predispositions:

- The artery and arteriole walls have a tendency to thicken and harden, a process known as arteriosclerosis. Oxygen and other nutrients carried by the blood have difficulty passing through the walls to reach the organs;
- The dermis lacks elastin and collagen. *Yellow rectangles* who smoke or go out without protection from the sun's ultraviolet rays may see their skin age very quickly. The skin can become saggy and wrinkled, and detach itself from the underlying muscles;
- The lack of oxygen on one hand, and of elastin and collagen on the other, result in the rapid aging not only of the skin, but of all the other organs as well;
- The adrenal glands are weak.

When *yellow rectangles* become imbalanced, they can be prone to the development of numerous disorders:

- Arthritis and osteoarthritis;
- Dilation of the capillary vessels (telangiectasia) caused by overexposure to sunlight, smoking and the lack of elastin and collagen;
- Neurological problems;
- Strokes;
- Tumors.

Because there is a great demand placed on their nervous systems, they may develop attention-deficit disorder at a very young age. It is important to monitor their adrenaline levels because of their susceptibility to chronic stress. They may also be candidates for irritable bowel syndrome and hypoglycemia. If they are vegans and their diet is too strict, they could suffer from insufficient intakes of protein, B-group vitamins and iron. As a result, they could experience periods of anemia and serious fatigue.

In summary, just like *green squares, yellow rectangles* have a tendency towards:

- Adrenal insufficiency
- Alzheimer's disease
- Anemia
- Anxiety
- Arteriosclerosis
- Attention-deficit disorder (ADD)
- Cancer
- Carpal tunnel syndrome
- Cystic acne
- Eczema
- Expressions wrinkles
- Fibrosis
- Fibrous cellulite
- Fibrous tumors
- Hepatitis
- Hypoglycemia
- Insomnia
- Irritable bowel syndrome
- Keloids
- Low blood pressure
- Milia (tiny whiteheads)
- Multiple sclerosis
- Osteoarthritis
- Osteoporosis
- Psoriasis
- Stretch marks

The *White Circle*

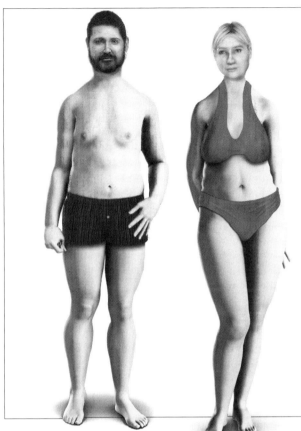

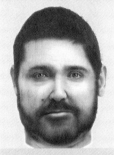

Has anyone ever told you that your skin is "like a baby's skin"?

Do you feel that your body is mostly made up of curves and round shapes?

Does your chin take up the largest portion of your face?

Physical traits

The lower zone of the face is predominant. The jawline is broad. A *white circle* will often have a double chin. The face appears round from either the front or the side. The entire body is fairly round.

Bones and muscles

The *white circle* has a large frame and big muscles. We are not talking here about someone frail or thin. The bones and muscles are not visible. *White circles* become obese if they are not on a permanent diet.

Why? For two specific reasons:

1 The hypodermis, the skin layer situated just under the dermis and epidermis, contains a large number of fat cells;

2 Under the epidermis, the cells of the dermis and the hypo-dermis are surrounded by more water (interstitial fluid) than normal.

It is this accumulation of fat and water that hides the shape of any adjacent structures.

The cheeks are round. The lips are as full as a *red oval's,* only not as firm.

The shoulders droop and the chest, in men as in women, is fleshy and broad. Viewed in profile, *white circles* display a very distinctive physical trait: the roundness of their stomachs seems to emanate right from the solar plexus. Because of this chronic edema, the shape of their thorax cannot be distinguished. Their bodies are pear-shaped. The two pairs of floating ribs (the 11th and 12th) cannot be seen at all. If these individuals try to locate the ends of these ribs with their thumbs, they will have difficulty finding them, as the layer of tissue covering them is too thick.

The waist is not visible, and the legs are large and heavy. There is no shape to their ankles, and their wrists are thickset. In sum, the tendency towards edema and toxin retention is pronounced and contributes to the roundness of their entire structure.

Skin and circulation

The skin is soft and pleasant to touch. It resembles the skin of a baby. The skin is mainly opaline-white with a gray overtone. A *white circle's* skin can have a pink undertone. It is easy to distinguish a pink-skinned *red oval* from a pink-skinned *white circle.* If you pinch the skin (dermis) on the forearm to try to lift it up, two things will happen: either it will lift, or it will not. If the skin does lift up, the person is a *white circle;* if it does not, the person is a *red oval.* It is impossible to lift the skin of a *red oval* and roll it between your fingers, whereas you can do that with the skin of a *white circle.* Note that in the case of *yellow rectangles* and *green squares,* it is the epidermal layer that lifts up.

Temperature and perspiration

When you touch the skin of a *white circle,* it can feel either warm or cold. The skin of an individual who is imbalanced will always be clammy. This is because the lymphatic system and internal organs (liver and kidneys) are doing a poor job of eliminating toxins. As a result, the only way for toxins to leave the body is through perspiration and secretions.

The tendency towards edema and toxin retention is pronounced and contributes to the roundness of their entire structure.

The skin is soft and pleasant to touch. It resembles the skin of a baby.

Body shape questionnaire
White circle

By now, you will all be eager to learn what your body type is. This quick questionnaire consists of a series of yes/no questions about the physical traits that characterize each shape. There are 10 for each shape, 40 in all.

Remember that fat is not what is important. Pay attention to the bone structure and the muscles. If the hormonal system is unbalanced, it will give rise to round shapes. Knowing that, be aware of your subject's age and hormonal balance (pregnancies, menopause, endropause, etc.).

Start by reading the whole questionnaire through. When you have finished , go back to the beginning and then begin answering the questions. Score your answers as follows:
- ❖ Write 1 if your answer is yes.
- ❖ Write 0 if your answer is no.
- ❖ If you find yourself hesitating, write 0, as if the answer were no.
- ❖ If you answer yes to one element in a series, write 1.

After working through the questions in the section for each shape, add up the points for that section and compare all the totals. You will find by the end that one shape will have received more points than the others, and this will be your predominant shape.

A few words of advice:

- ❖ Do not worry: answering with a 0 does not mean you fall short in any way; it is your genetic inheritance!
- ❖ Similarly, writing 1 is not necessarily a reason to be proud!
- ❖ Do not be too hard on yourself. This is an activity to enjoy, not a final exam!
- ❖ Remember that you are measuring yourself. Never compare yourself to another person.
- ❖ If you are carrying a few extra pounds, do not worry. Fat does not count.
- ❖ Identifying what we are is a lot more difficult than identifying what we are not. So if you are unsure in any way about a question, I suggest you try a process of elimination. Just move on to the next question—or the one after that—until you find one that you know you can answer with a 1. If you are ready, let's go!

White circle	
1.	Has anyone ever told you that your skin is "as soft as a baby's skin"?
2.	Do you find your body curvaceous? Are the lines of your body rounded?
3.	Do you have a tendency to put on weight easily?
4.	Does the lower part of your face stand out?
5.	Do you have drooping shoulders?
6.	Are you big-chested?
7.	Does your waist seem large and rounded?
8.	Are your legs big and solid? Do they sometimes seem heavy?
9.	Do you sometimes experience cold sweats?
10.	In the morning when you wake up, are your legs sometimes swollen?
Total out of 10:	

Now compare the results for each of the four sets of questions. The highest score indicates your predominant shape, the shape you were born with.

You did not choose this shape. It came to you hand in hand with a number of genetic predispositions and with its advantages and disadvantages. In the second part of the book you can read how, through your own choices and decisions, you can make your strengths work for you, while compensating for any weaknesses.

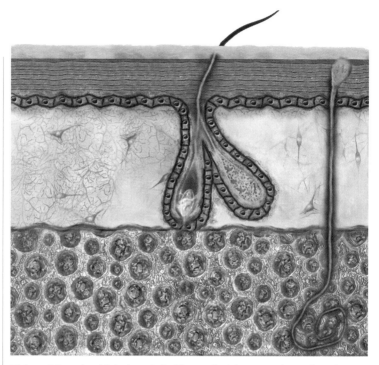

Thin epidermis, thick dermis infiltrated with water, hypodermis contains a large number of fat cells.

Metabolism

White circles' metabolisms are slow. Everything they eat or drink seems to accumulate in their bodies. They cannot control their hydrostatic equilibrium, partly because their tissue accumulates far more water than is necessary and partly because they have poor pancreatic function. They do not produce enough bile salt, which interferes with the digestion of fats and sugars.

They use a great amount of energy to digest, and this explains why they invariably feel sleepy after a big meal. If you are giving a conference around two o'clock in the afternoon, do not be offended if a *white circle* drops off to sleep while you are speaking. They are not being impolite; it is simply a way of saving energy over which they have no control!

Nervous system

They do not experience a lot of stress.

In *white circles,* there is not a lot of demand placed on the central nervous system and the sympathetic nervous system. They do not experience a lot of stress. They are not pumped full of adrenaline like *green squares* and *yellow rectangles.* However, do not be under the false impression that this means they are slow to grasp things. In conversation, they are extremely attentive to details and take great care to fully understand any practical or concrete matters.

If they have a long list of things to accomplish, they will work for longer, without accelerating their rhythm, to be sure to finish. The fact is, they have confidence in themselves and are comfortable with their pace, so why should they rush?

❖

Sumo

Since the beginning of my career, I have had the good fortune to travel the world giving conferences on skin and skin disorders. From the Far East to South America, passing through the most exotic places you can imagine, I have demonstrated the principles found in this book—with the obstinacy of a *green square* and the passion that animates a *red oval!* The world, in all its diversity, was waiting for this suburban girl that I was to discover.

In the middle of this professional and personal whirlwind, I found myself on a plane from Japan to Montreal—a long, 18-hour flight! We were over the Pacific, and I looked up mechanically at the movie that was playing. I was literally stupefied to see, for the first time in my life, sumo wrestlers. Although sumo wrestling was the national sport of Japan, and these athletes were venerated as demi-gods, I had never witnessed this, not even in photos. You can imagine my astonishment.

Seeing how I was taken aback, the passenger in the seat next to me set about explaining the rudiments of this combat sport as well as its significance in her culture. This elegant Japanese woman continued by explaining that the bodies of the rikishi, or wrestlers, were conditioned by selecting certain foods over others to ensure weight gain.

What completely astounded me about this spectacle was not so much the sight of these enormous men, garbed only in what appeared to me to be G-strings, fighting in the center of a delirious crowd of onlookers, but the fact that what I was witnessing was a sport in which the participating athletes were all predominantly *white circles*.

Once I had absorbed this, I explained my passion for body typology to the woman and we whiled away the hours in an uninterrupted flow of conversation. Far from being uniquely a question of diet, the training of a sumo wrestler hinges, in the first place, on genetic predisposition. The athlete must be a dominant *white circle* before subjecting himself to such a regime. *Yellow rectangles* could gorge themselves with as much high calorie foods as they wished, yet they would never be able to stand up to a *white circle*. They would be pummeled into the ground on the very first attack.

❖

Psychological traits

White circles live for their families and close friends, not for themselves.

They jump to conclusions, sometimes too quickly, and they make assumptions about things based on only one or two examples. In the same way, they are quick to form opinions about people. They take very little time—sometimes not nearly enough—to comment on something: if a *white circle* reads a text you have just written, within no time he or she will find fault with it and suggest a number of modifications. They can do this without much difficulty because they are so absolutely sure of themselves. *White circles* can be as stubborn as *green squares.*

What is important for them is not scientific truth, but emotional truth and human relations.

In conversation, they like to discuss the news they have heard on the radio, seen on television, or read in the newspapers. They will report on the opinions of well-known personalities from the world of politics or other fields. Generally, the fields of research, science and advanced technologies hold no interest for them. What is important for them is not scientific truth, but emotional truth and human relations. They get involved in causes that make sense and are just.

You will find *white circles* running support group committees, working in the caring professions, often in hospitals, and then volunteering even more of their time in these institutions once their workday is done. They are pillars of their communities, volunteering their time for various activities, schools and clubs. Saving the world gives meaning to their lives.

Happy, smiling and ready to help, they would do anything for you. They will worry about you even if you do not ask for help. They truly have your best interests at heart. What you own is of no interest to them. They do not envy anybody and have no desire for anybody to envy them. Their temperaments perfectly suit their inclination to serve and to be practical.

It is interesting to note, however, that they are by no means slaves to their good deeds. In fact, they are very independent. They love to travel, planning trips well in advance. They anticipate any and all circumstances and leave nothing behind: first aid kit, extra batteries, international electrical adapter, UV-protection cream, mosquito repellent, etc. They evaluate all possible eventualities and, come the day of departure, they are well and truly ready for anything.

They are extremely generous, asking nothing in return but an ear to listen to them. They talk a lot and express themselves easily. They have a need to talk, to tell stories, to offer advice. Moreover, they are such good conversationalists, cheerful and animated, with opinions about everything, that nobody dares to interrupt them! *Green squares* say that *white circles* force them to spend far too much time on the phone!

In a crisis, they are extremely effective. They never fear for themselves, and they remain calm. Their concern is for others, and they will come quickly when their help is needed. They can endure nightmarish situations, yet still sleep well at night. In general, they are excellent caregivers to the very sick, to those whose suffering is unbearable to most people. And once their work is done, they will take full advantage of their time off and wake up the next morning full of optimism. *White circles* take life one day at a time and plan for the future so as not to leave others in difficulty. As long as they get along well with their loved ones, life is good. In short, they live for their families.

White circles dress comfortably, not ostentatiously or flamboyantly. They dress to be able to do what they have to do, not to be noticed. They do not depart from the norm, make waves, or attract attention; they dress sensibly. This does not mean that they have any hesitation about expressing their opinions. They simply have no wish to rock the boat. They believe that consensus is always the best strategy, and abhor conflict and arguments. They never express anger and rely on patience and time to get what they want. They would rather go without something than be demanding or complain.

They are eminently practical. If you were building a house and you invited a friend who is a *white circle* to look at the construction in progress, that friend would give you lots of extremely sound, albeit unsolicited, advice. Friends who are *white circles* feel that the job cannot possibly progress without them; you may even feel like asking them to mind their own business.

Nevertheless, it would be in your interest to hear what they had to say. They may be quicker and more observant than you in perceiving a potential danger for children. They may note something that could be built in such a way as to be more convenient for the elderly or those with reduced mobility. *White circles* do not care about having praise heaped on them for the good advice they offer; saving the world is their just reward! They have a formidable sense of what is practical. They stick their noses everywhere precisely because they anticipate problems and accidents. Their cautiousness and benevolence are at the root of the outpouring of their good advice. To them, a house must be safe (just try to stop a *white circle* from talking if he or she has detected a potential danger!) and practical for the entire family.

White circles feel good about their bodies. Being plump does not worry them in the slightest. Let people talk, for all they care! They would be completely comfortable strolling through a nudist colony, curves and all. Even so, they are not insensitive and would be hurt if they knew you were talking about them behind their backs.

Although they do not like sports, they love to go for walks.

Although they do not like sports (they "don't have the time"), they love to go for walks.

They are attracted to professions that require precision, patience, or meticulousness: accountant, auditor, or financial analyst. Other occupations to which they might be drawn include those that require availability and dedication: nurse, EMT (Emergency Medical Technician), social worker, family service agent, daycare worker. If you are looking for a volunteer, you won't find a better person.

They like to restore balance. They are peacemakers and they seek the company of those who make peace. They loathe having to fight for their rights. They will not make a fuss in public, but have no qualms about pouring their hearts out in writing or to someone close to them. But do not think you can just walk over a *white circle:* they are tenacious and will persevere until they get what is coming to them.

White circles do not often go to salons or spas.

White circles do not often go to salons or spas. If they have to go on the recommendation of a doctor (to alleviate backache or to improve lymphatic circulation), they may agree to have a massage or pressotherapy perhaps. They may eventually even consent to a pedicure, as they dislike bending over! They certainly will not go to be pampered. There has to be a therapeutic objective to their visit.

White circles are full of energy in the morning and should use that time for their necessary tasks. If, on the other hand, they are on vacation, or are still teenagers, they love to sleep late.

Although they are able to dispense all manner of practical and sound advice, they cannot help but feel that they never quite get it right themselves. They are perpetually worried that someone hite circles are always ready to wake up early to attend a workshop to improve their helping skills. In fact, they will be the first to arrive and the last to leave. Red ovals, on the other hand, would feel as though they were missing out on something in the conference next door. As far as green squares are concerned, they may arrive late but would listen attentively for the first 10 minutes or so. They would take notes but, deeming the content not up to their level, would soon let their attention drift elsewhere. Yellow rectangles would want everything validated. They would ask a slew of questions, appearing terribly learned to all those participating.

✛

might reproach them for having forgotten something or made a mistake. As a result, they are self-effacing and prefer to stay in the shadows.

The past holds special meaning for them, and they delight in recounting the same funny or sad anecdotes, based on their experiences. They have infallible memories and never forget a birthday. They decorate their houses with loving care during the holidays and are full of ideas when it comes to family birthdays and other festive occasions. They go in for celebrations, invocations, costumes, toasts and all rituals that honor friendship, joy and peace in the family or among friends. They are extremely loyal and sincere. Once they bestow their friendship and confidence on you, you can count on them for life!

Assets and genetic predispositions

Physical assets

White circles are not lacking in physical assets. Their skin is as soft as a baby's, milky and full, with not a wrinkle to be seen. Their general health is good. Their whole appearance exudes well-being. They have good circulation and their tissues are well-oxygenated and well-balanced.

Genetic predispositions

White circles struggle throughout their lives to maintain balanced hydrostatic pressure. Their bodies accumulate fluid and toxins and their tendency towards edema is what is so striking in them. Their lymphatic circulation is particularly slow. The valves that retain lymph fluids are weak and slow, resulting in poor drainage of the lymph fluids.

Because of water retention, they are prone to high blood pressure and venous insufficiency. They are often troubled by related conditions including arteriosclerosis, the risk of strokes (blood clots) and cardiac arrhythmia. Their adrenal glands do not produce enough adrenalin. Contrary to *yellow rectangles* or *green squares,* their parasympathetic nervous system affects them considerably, resulting in hyperextensibility of the joints and a permanent air of calm.

Toxins build up in the body. Wastes are not easily transformed to allow for proper elimination. They tend to accumulate in the connective tissues and in the muscles. This produces the *white circles'* rotund shape. *White circles* have poor muscle tone.

White circles tend to be chubby. If they do not watch their diets constantly, they will suffer from obesity. This has nothing to do with overeating, but with their inability to properly transform sugars and fats due to a poorly functioning pancreas. They do not produce enough bile salts.

When they form cellulite, it is not the hard, fibrous cellulite, but the soft (hydric) cellulite from water retention, which is much easier to treat than its counterpart. Because of their excess weight and their bodies' inability to properly regulate water, they often develop arthritis.

Lastly, they have a predisposition to developing fibromyalgia.

Like *red ovals,* they have a tendency towards:
- Angina
- Allergies
- Arrhythmia
- Asthma
- Blood clots (strokes, thrombosis, pulmonary embolism)
- Diabetes
- Elephantiasis
- Fibromyalgia
- Gout
- High blood pressure
- High cholesterol (high levels of LDL, or low-density lipoprotein)

- Inflammatory arthritis
- Kidney disease
- Lymphedema
- Palpitations
- Chubbiness
- Rosacea
- Soft (hydric) cellulite
- Thyroid gland imbalance
- Venous insufficiency
- Weak immune system

Exercise 3.
Face value: shape and proportion

For this exercise, you will need four or five magazines and a few felt markers. Avoid fashion magazines because the models you see in them will be predominantly yellow rectangles and green squares. That is right; most of today's fashion models fall into those two categories. Each period throughout history considers the physical traits of one type or another to be universal ideals of beauty.

First, leaf through the magazines to select about 20 photographs. Try to find full-page photos in which you can see the models' faces from the front or slightly in profile. Mark the pages that you select with a paper clip, a yellow self-stick note, or, even better, cut the pages right out and put them in a file folder.

Look at the faces one by one without rushing your analysis. Because predominant skin tones can be altered by makeup, computer re-touching, or printing procedures, you are simply going to consider the shape and proportions of the face for this exercise.

Examine each of your chosen subjects and answer these questions:

❖ When you look at the contours of the face, does it seem to you more round (ample) or square (angular)? On the photo, draw a " ∨" for the ones that are ample and a "‿" for the ones that are angular. Sort them into the two categories before going on to the next question.

❖ Separate the face into three sections with dotted lines: the forehead, the eyes and cheeks and the lower portion. If one section is predominant, mark a " * " on it.

❖ Is the chin round or square? Is there a double chin or is the shape of the chin ill-defined? Are the cheekbones prominent? Does the hairline recede in a pronounced "V" to expose the forehead? Draw curves or angles beside the face to point out the most striking trait

❖ Have another look at each subject and decide
whether the shapes, proportions and particularities of the
face indicate the predominance of one type. Make a note of
your answer.

You will soon see that several of your subjects clearly belong to one
type or another. For the others, the analysis will not be conclusive. Do
not forget, however, that this is only a partial analysis, using only the
facial characteristics. If you have been able to conclusively identify
just a few faces, then the exercise has been a success. The goal of each
of these exercises is to improve your powers of observation.

Duration: 60 minutes

Exercise 4.
A body of evidence: shape and proportion

Over the course of these first few exercises, you have probably begun to realize that seeing and observing are, in fact, quite distinct from one another. In our day-to-day lives, we only notice what we need in order to go about our activities. The more you invest in the analysis of body typology, the more your perception will improve. You will see things more keenly; you will notice more detail. Just like a muscle that you work for the first time, it takes an effort at the beginning. And just as you can firm up your muscles with the effort you put in, so can you strengthen your perception. Today we will look at the shapes and proportions of the body to decide whether they belong to the ample family or the angular family.

❖ Look at the angle made between the head and shoulders. Are the shoulders round and somewhat puffy (red oval)? Are they square and muscular (green square)? Does the person look bony, narrow and square (yellow rectangle)? Do the shoulders droop, giving the person the shape of a bottle (white circle)?

Here is a generalized image to help you distinguish between the two families. Imagine making an incision in the top of a person's forehead and pouring in liters of water between the skin and the bones. Visualize the water running down the body to the feet. In those belonging to the ample family, the water would accumulate, producing round shapes and curves, and the muscles would swell. In those belonging to the angular family, it would drain out, and the angles of the bones and muscles would be visible.

Detailed morphological evaluation

By now, you should have a good overview of the different body types. Has reading through the leading questions for each type given you an idea of which type you are? If so, the questionnaire has put you on the track of your dominant type.

However, if you find that you are still undecided, there is no need to worry. It does not matter if you cannot identify your type for the time being. In fact, there are very few pure *red ovals, green squares, yellow rectangles,* or *white circles.* This is what the evaluation questionnaire was designed to show.

In most of us, one dominant type does show through, but it comes with a whole series of secondary characteristics belonging to other types. This explains why we hesitate over some of our answers. So unless it is blatantly obvious, try not to leap at the first type that seems to resemble you a bit; even worse, make sure you do not go for the type you would like to be!

It can be quite a surprise for most people when they hear their recorded voice or watch themselves on a video. How many of us exclaim in amazement, "Is that really how I sound?" Our friends never fail to reply, "Well yes, that's exactly what you sound like!" No one said it would be easy to watch, observe and evaluate ourselves. You need to be able to distance yourself quite a bit in order to be able to look at yourself objectively. So if you really want to master the morphological evaluation techniques properly, I suggest practicing on other people. The more people you evaluate, the better-practiced your eye will be in allowing you to do an impartial self-evaluation.

This is the section in which you will get the first chance to measure yourself by working through the same type evaluation sequence I use, which I teach to doctors, medical students, nurses, estheticians and therapists all over the world. For each point of the evaluation, you will find many references throughout the

You will get the first chance to measure yourself by working through the same type evaluation sequence I use.

book. So please feel free to look back to some of the earlier sections in which some of these points were first mentioned.

Your first impression may well be that the evaluation seems a little complicated, and, in fact, I have to agree with you. You cannot learn to do a good body type evaluation in a mere five minutes. But I promise you that your patience will be rewarded, and, after a little practice, you will be amazed at how well you are doing. To guide you through the process, I have devised 12 simple and enjoyable exercises, which have already begun to help you grasp the main aspects of the evaluation. These exercises can be found spread throughout this book. As we take you through the observation process, you will soon start to appreciate not only how easy it is becoming, but also just how much valuable information it can yield.

The evaluation sequence

Before we start, there are a few ground rules that will help you avoid making some common mistakes.

- Relax. Take a few deep breaths. Stress limits your powers of observation.
- Allow yourself to be curious. Curiosity encourages concentration and helps you to suspend judgment.
- Do not jump to conclusions when you see lots of fat!
- Very few people are one pure type.
- Base your evaluation on the person's physical characteristics, not on their psychological characteristics. We are not only what genetics has made us. Just as much as our genetic inheritance, lifestyle choices, values, emotional make-up, family and social environments, the culture we were born into, as well as our own past, all combine to make us who we are.

Be systematic. Learning the methodology properly means following the evaluation one step at a time, starting at the beginning and finishing at the end. And the more rigorous your evaluation, the better your results will be. Afterwards, should you wish, you can always go back and give additional attention to some points and less attention to others. This is exactly how I proceed in an evaluation.

Ample or angular?
(Evaluation part one)

Each of the four body shapes can be divided into two classes: ample and angular. Start by identifying which of these two main classes the individual belongs to. Then you will be able to be more specific. To determine the class, we look at two things:

- Shape,
- The skin color palette.

You are trying to form an overall impression at this stage, rather than looking for details. Do not worry at this point about deciding once and for all that a person is ample or angular. Your first impression can always be revised.

Shape: general evaluation

Red ovals and *white circles* give a general impression of roundness. *Green squares* and *yellow rectangles,* however, are quite the opposite. At first glance, it is the angles of their bodies that strike an observer. If the person is a little on the heavy side, do not let the mass of adipose tissue mislead you into classifying them as ample: a *green square* can be overweight too.

- Look at the subject overall.
- Look at the body generally—hips, waist and shoulders. Do you get an impression of roundness or do you see angles?
- Look at the general shape of the face. Is the face rounded (ample) or rather narrow (angular)?

Skin color: the palette

Despite the great variety of different skin tones that exist, do not forget that all color is essentially a mixture of three primary colors. It makes no difference that someone has a very white Scandinavian skin or an almost ebony African skin. Behind the light-dark scale of skin tone, one palette of color will always predominate.

Amples have skin that falls into the red-white palette, and angulars have skin in the green-yellow range. Have a look in the section dealing with colors to see some of the color palettes in different skin tones for amples and angulars.

- Look for some bare skin. Perhaps the arms or the lower neck. Do not just look at the face. Try to look at skin that has not been exposed to the sun. Overall, in which palette would you place this skin

It can be easier to decide the predominant skin color from a distance. From too close up our eye is distracted by details. Look at the section on color to see photos of predominant green-yellow skin and red-white skin in different tones.

These first two observations will tell you what class the person belongs to, which you will probably have been able to judge from your overall impression. Class can be very marked or it can be quite subtle. Now it is time to go a little deeper in your examination to determine the predominant type. To do this you will be looking out for distinctive signs.

Observing type
(Evaluation part two)

The next step is to identify your subject's predominant type by using a more detailed version of the criteria we saw in the last section.

Body shape and proportions

- ❖ Take a good full-length look at the person. In order to be able to judge proportions, the subject should be standing up. You cannot very well compare the length of someone's legs to the rest of the body when they are seated!
- ❖ Observe their body shape:
  - Are the shoulders rounded (*oval*), sloping (*circle*), or square (*square*) and bony (*rectangle*)?
  - Look at the triceps muscle when the arm is relaxed. (It is the muscle at the back of the arm that goes between the shoulder and the elbow) Is it clear-cut (*square*), naturally rounded (*oval*), long and delicate (*rectangle*), or hardly visible among the general fullness of the upper arm (*circle*)?
  - In relation to the hips, is the waist slender (*square*), narrow (*rectangle*), short (*oval*), or wide (*circle*)?
  - Look at the chest. Is it rounded (*oval*), obvious and well-defined (*square*)? Drooping and not very present (*rectangle*)? Large and heavy (*circle*)?
  - What about the shape of the buttocks? Are they high and rounded (*oval*), or carried low (*square*)? Are they hardly even noticeable (*rectangle*), or are they much fuller and not so well-defined (*circle*)?

- Observe the thighs in the same way as the triceps.
- Take a quick look at the calves. How are they built? How muscular are they? Is there any sign of swelling around the ankle, foot or, indeed, in the leg generally (*circle*)?

Face shape and proportions

The shapes and proportions of our faces often mirror those of our bodies. It is thought that they echo each other. However, this can sometimes be misleading.

- What shape of face does your subject have? Is it oval (*red oval*), square (*green square*), rectangular (*yellow rectangle*), or round (*white circle*)?
- Does one part of the face seem to take up more space: maybe the forehead (*yellow rectangle*), the centre (*red oval*), or the lower half (*white circle*)?
- Look at the forehead. Does it fit with the rest of the face and look square (*green square*)? Is it wide (*white circle*), heart-shaped (*yellow rectangle*), or well-proportioned (*green square*)?
- Observe the middle part of the face. Does the subject have high cheekbones (*red oval*)?
- Observe the lower part of the face. What is the jawline like? Can you see the beginnings of a double chin (*white circle*)?
- Look at the lips. Are they fleshy with good blood circulation (*red oval*), well-defined (*green square*), thin (*yellow rectangle*), full and poorly defined with inadequate circulation (*white circle*)?

Specific skin tone

- Look at the range of facial skin tones.
- Observe the skin on the neck and on the top of the chest, preferably in places where the skin is usually protected from the sun.
- Look at any bare skin you can see. Look at the skin on the legs. Your subject may be wearing pants, but see if you can get a glimpse of the foot above the shoe.
- Grasp the wrist. Turn the arm over in both directions to get a good look at the inside and outside of the forearm. This will give you a better idea of the skin's full range of tone.

Skin characteristics

- Test the capillary return. Press the inner side of the forearm hard using two or three fingers. Watch how the skin loses color; look for the color to return and see how long it takes. The capillary return test can be repeated on the upper part of the chest.

- ❖ Pinch the skin of the forearm between your thumb and fingers. The pinch test allows you to test for a number of factors at the same time.
  - Is there an infiltration of liquid (ample)?
  - Is the dermis firmly attached to the epidermis (ample), or do feel that the skin is loose (angular)?
  - Is the epidermis thick (angular) or thin (ample)?
  - Does the skin feel elastic (angular) or taut (ample)?
- ❖ Test the temperature of the skin. Is it warm (ample) or cold (angular)?
- ❖ Does the skin feel clammy (ample) or dry (angular)?

Anyone who is interested in skin health and care will naturally also be looking out for the following:

- ❖ Is the skin soft (*circle*)? Does it have a smooth texture (ample) or is it rough (angular)?
- ❖ Do you see dead skin flaking on the surface (angular)?
- ❖ Are there any hyperpigmentation spots (angular)? Can you see signs of redness (telangiectasia) (*oval*), or any other abnormalities?

Be aware that skin can be tricky to observe. Foundation, blushes, other cosmetics and aesthetic treatments all mask the skin's natural look. People find ways of cheating on nature. Fortunately, the forearms and upper chest area never receive as much attention and are good places to see the skin in its natural state.

Refine your evaluation
(Evaluation part three)

Particularities

Note any signs that will point you in a particular direction. You might see people who look like obvious *red ovals* until you notice that they have swollen ankles or feet, which makes you think *white circles.*

Key questions

The key questions are those that are going to sway your decision, by using a process of elimination, in favor of one type over another. This is because these questions are always geared to understanding how your subject's physiology will react to a particular situation. They will give an indication of how we can expect the person's body to react and change over time. Until now, we have been making evaluations that are more static.

1. Do you sweat easily (*red oval*)?
2. Do you blush or turn red easily (*red oval*)?
3. Are your hands and feet cold (*green square*)?
4. Are you cold all the time (*yellow rectangle*)?

General psychological portrait

In the first part of the book, we gave a broad explanation of the predispositions of temperament that are typical of *red ovals, green squares, yellow rectangles* and *white circles.* At the outset, it was stated that morphological evaluations cannot be carried out based on a person's attitudes, or psychological characteristics alone. Keep in mind that skin tone is, in fact, the principal indicator of temperament.

This being said, since the evaluation is almost complete at this stage, there is no reason now not to look at some character traits alongside our objective observations. If the character traits confirm our analysis, then all is well and good. If not, it will encourage us to try another direction and to check if anything has been overlooked. Some character traits develop with age.

So go ahead and ask questions. Get to know your subjects. You may already know what their jobs are, whether they have families and what they do in their spare time. Ask people about their personal and professional lives. Generally, it is fairly easy to get people to talk about themselves.

A proper evaluation is the result of careful study. It is not a guessing game. I cannot emphasize enough how important it is to keep your eyes open. Every individual is unique and deserves to be observed thoroughly. During our analysis, things can temporarily become a little unclear, or, at times, we will not be able to see into which group a characteristic fits. It is at such moments that even more rigor is called for, and we must be careful to proceed with even more caution. Hasty conclusions invariably lead to inappropriate treatments or to an unsound cure. The opposite is also true. When you work with the true nature, the deep essence of each individual, however complex this may be, the results will be just as good as you could ever hope for.

A proper evaluation is the result of careful study. It is not a guessing game.

When you work with the true nature, the deep essence of each individual, the results will be just as good as you could ever hope for.

The morphological evaluation: points of reference

1 Determine the class
- General evaluation of the shape of the body and face
- Determine the palette: yellow / green or white / red

2 Determine the type
- Body shape and proportions
- Face shape and proportions
- Specific skin tone

3 Refine the evaluation
- Particularities
- Key questions
- General psychological portrait

Body

	Red oval	*Green square*	*Yellow rectangle*	*White circle*
Shoulders	Round.	Square.	Bony.	Sloping.
Triceps	Rounded.	Sculpted.	Long and delicate.	Imperceptible.
Waist	Not well-defined.	Defined.	Narrow.	Large.
Chest	Round and high. In women, a plunging cleavage.	Medium. In women, breasts nicely separated. Clavicles barely discernible.	Drooping, not very present.	Drooping, large and heavy.
Buttocks	High and rounded.	Pronounced.	Small.	Large and round.
Calves	Rounded.	Sculpted.	Thin.	Swelling at the ankle.
Proportions	All curves. Rotund and solid.	Perfect proportions. Broad shoulders, slender waist, elongated legs.	Tall and thin. Elongated trunk and arms, narrow shoulders.	Big and heavy legs. Round solar plexus.
Muscles	Rounded and bulbous.	Well-formed, well-defined, sculpted.	Long, slender, ill-defined.	Hidden, barely visible, lacking muscle tone.
Bones	Big bones.	Medium.	Light and frail, visible under the skin, ribs and pelvic bones very noticeable.	Big bones, hidden.

Face

	Red oval	*Green square*	*Yellow rectangle*	*White circle*
Shape	Oval.	Square, even if long.	Rectangular or triangular.	Round.
Traits	Ill-defined.	Well-defined and pronounced, clearly visible nose folds.	Pronounced.	Ill-defined.
Proportions	Cheekbones predominant.	Balanced.	Forehead predominant.	Lower half of face predominant.
Chin	Oval.	Square, straight.	Pointed.	Double chin.
Lips	Full.	Shapely.	Thin, corners of the mouth turned down.	Full, not well-defined.

ANTI-AGING · THE CURE

Skin

	Red oval	Green square	Yellow rectangle	White circle
Tone	Rosy.	Olive.	Yellow.	White.
Epidermis	Thin.	Thick.	Very thick.	Thin.
Dermis	Thick, well-vascularized and well-oxygenated.	Thin, poorly vascularized.	Very thin, poorly vascularized and very poorly oxygenated.	Thick, infiltrated with water. Hypodermis contains a large number of fat cells and water.
Collagen	High.	Low.	Low to medium-low.	Medium.
Texture	Moist.	Normal.	Rough, granular.	Soft.
Temperature	Warm or normal.	Normal, cold extremities when under stress.	Cold or normal.	Clammy or normal.
Perspiration	Abundant.	Hands and feet sweat when under stress. .	Very little.	When unbalanced, skin becomes clammy.

Particular skin characteristics

	Red oval	Green square	Yellow rectangle	White circle
Scarring	Very good.	Poor.	Poor.	Good.
Predispositions	Areas of redness, rosacea, acne rosacea, melanoma. Rhinophyma.	Pigmentation spots, stretch marks, milia, eczema, psoriasis, oily or dry skin.	Hydrolipic imbalance, pigmentation spots stretch marks, milia, eczema, psoriasis, oily skin.	Accumulation of toxins, water infiltration, edema.
Type of cellulite	Hydric.	Fibrous.	Fibrous.	Hydric.
Vascularization	Venous insufficiency.	Normal.	Poorly vascularized.	Venous and lymphatic insufficiency.
Wrinkles	Few.	Expression wrinkles.	Wrinkles rapidly, wrinkles are pronounced, lack of muscle tone, skin tends to droop.	Few, baby-soft skin.
Sensitivity to the environment	Highly sensitive.	Normal.	Normal.	Highly sensitive.
Other	Well-oxygenated.	When tired, can develop a green tinge. Poorly-oxygenated.	Accumulation of dead skin, rough, can develop a gray tinge.	Water infiltration, soft and pleasant to touch.

Psychological profile

	Red oval	Green square	Yellow rectangle	White circle
Fundamental motivation	To be recognized.	To control.	To maintain routine.	To help family.
Relationship with others	Extroverted, easy conversationalist, wants to please, easily impassioned about things.	Extroverted, likes to be in control of a conversation.	Introverted, a follower, timid.	Introverted, talks a lot, cheerful.
Fundamental attitude	Tends towards social relationships, good humor, changeable, impulsive, energetic.	Action-oriented, tendency to become stressed.	Thoughtful, perpetually anxious, insecure.	Tends towards family or group relationships.
Call to action	Impulsive / reactive, works in fits and starts.	Plans according to objectives, workaholic.	Reactive, thoughtful, a creature of habit.	Perfectionist who works at own pace, can lack energy (due to a lack of adrenaline), tenacious.
Relationship with money	Likes to spend it.	Likes to make it, a negotiator, ambitious.	Likes to save it, thrifty.	Doesn't worry about it, spends it on loved ones.
Tasks	One task at a time.	Multitasking is normal way of operating, likes to perform several tasks at once.	Likes to be involved in several tasks at once.	At own pace, one task at a time.
Attitude to time	Lives from day to day, dreaming about the future.	Lives in the future, organizes today with tomorrow in view.	Lives in the past.	Lives in the present, has foresight.
Reactions and characteristic attitudes	Quick-tempered, becomes as quickly impassioned as disenchanted, enjoys being complimented, impulsive, impressionable.	Autonomous, independent, stubborn, skeptical, extremist, demanding, egocentric, likes to stand out from the crowd, honest, a perfectionist.	Loyal and dependable, responsible, enjoys learning, opportunistic, curious, often illogical.	Helpful, generous, quick to judge people, keeps a cool head, practical, stubborn.
Other traits	Enjoys good food, fashionable, lacks self-esteem.	Enjoys that which is exclusive, competitive, looks after own self-interests, dominant.	Enjoys nature and animals, plays sports, disciplined, inventive, imaginative, competitive, a sore loser, nervous and timid, has trouble completing projects.	Sense of detail, precise, keeps a cool head, generous, practical, loathes sports, good, honest, dependable, has foresight, lives for others.

The cure

Introduction to the Four Areas

Traditional Chinese medicine, Ayurvedic medicine and Greco-Roman medicine all agree on one thing: that nature cures disease. The role of the physician is to help the sick to recognize and abide by their true nature. More precisely, the physician helps those who are sick to stop fighting their true nature and to discover the lifestyle, exercises and foods that are going to lessen their weaknesses and strengthen their natural immunity.

Hippocrates put it directly: "One has to be well-informed about the nature of man in his totality, to know what man is fundamentally and to distinguish truly the component parts that predominate in him. For he who does not know about the fundamental makeup of man and what rules his body can never make useful prescriptions." (See Hippocratic Oath)

In the first part of this book, you learned about the physical and psychological traits that characterize each body type. You have also been able to complete the quick questionnaires to determine your own form and color and, in doing so, determine your predominant type. You have been introduced to our evaluation method and the first series of observation exercises has helped you sharpen your perceptions. There will be more exercises to do before you have finished reading this book. Once you have completed 12 of them, it would be a good idea to revise your auto-evaluation.

Having become aware of your assets and inclinations, in the second part of this book you are going to learn how to use what you have learned about your type to help you age better. You are going to take preventive measures to protect yourself from the diseases that you are naturally at risk of contracting, and you are going to stop wasting energy fighting against your true nature.

As you know only too well, we cannot turn back the clock. But by following your natural paths, you can directly influence the workings of the cells of your body. You are going to change your outward appearance by changing your interior. This change will take place gradually as you make little adjustments in four areas of everyday life. These adjustments will enable you to find the balance that lies at the heart of your anti-aging treatment.

The four areas that we are going to look at correspond to the four standard questions:

- Why should I exercise?
- What foods suit me best?
- How can I take care of my skin?
- Why should I take care of my relationships with other people?

First of all, some general comments.

Why should I exercise?

Exercise is good for you in all kinds of ways.

Oxygenation of the heart

Physical exercise keeps the circulatory system in good health. It brings oxygen to the heart and arteries. A well-oxygenated heart does its job well.

Oxygenation and nourishment of the whole body

By pumping blood through the arteries, exercise leads to oxygenation of all the tissues: skin, muscles, ligaments, bones and internal organs. This, in turn, means that food needed by tissue cells is delivered to them. In other words, exercise speeds up the rate at which the heart beats and thus the rate at which the blood delivers the oxygen and nutrients that cells need to survive.

By following your natural paths, you can directly influence the workings of the cells of your body.

Nourishing cells

Exercise has an effect on the basal metabolic rate and, thus, on the basic energy equation. This equation describes the transformation that takes place in our bodies to produce the energy our cells need. Nutrients are the components of food that have been digested and transformed into a form in which our cells can absorb them. On one side of the energy equation are the nutrients that will be transformed in the presence of oxygen, and on the other side are the products of this transformation.

Among these products is ATP (adenosine triphosphate), the biochemical compound that cells directly consume. ATP is the fuel that the body absolutely needs. All the other products of transformation—such as heat, carbon dioxide, water and waste—are either eliminated or recycled. According to the needs of the moment, for instance, some of the water produced is recycled while the rest is eliminated.

The basic metabolic equation is: nutrients (i.e., food) + oxygen (i.e., air) = adenosine triphosphate + carbonic acid + water + heat + waste.

As soon as the supply of oxygen goes up, so does the production of carbon dioxide, water and heat. Sweat serves to get rid of some of this water, wastes and heat.

The only signs of aging that people fear are the signs of premature aging. When you suffer from signs of premature aging and compare yourself to others who do not, you often feel like stopping the flow of time, even if you know that it is not possible.

Let time do its work, and let us do ours. Skin and other organs that are well-maintained, well-oxygenated and well-nourished easily regenerate their cells and preserve their functions for a very long time. When the marks of time do appear on a healthy body, they always appear together in a coherent way. In a healthy organism, the beauty of the whole is always preserved as time passes.

When metabolic reactions are working well, you do not see signs of accelerated aging. What you do see are signs of good health, and these signs gently and progressively evolve, always preserving their harmony.

The signs of accelerated aging are reversible: they can disappear if you find a lifestyle in which, once again, your body is well-exercised, well-oxygenated, well-nourished and relaxed. Of course, there are also surgical procedures, both invasive as well as non-invasive.

In a healthy organism, the beauty of the whole is always preserved as time passes.

The signs of accelerated aging are reversible: they can disappear if you find a lifestyle in which your body is well-exercised, well-oxygenated, well-nourished and relaxed.

Breathing and exercise

It is well known that physical exercise accelerates the breathing rate.

For some 15 years, specialists in physical training have known that when breathing is slow and regular, the heart rhythm tends to synchronize with the breathing rhythm. The heart takes the regular rise and fall of the diaphragm as a reference and can adjust its rhythm to this beat. More precisely, it speeds up when the diaphragm falls and slows down when the diaphragm rises.

When these accelerations and decelerations become regular, the vagus nerve, which links the brain with the heart, transmits this good news to the brain, which then triggers two processes, both with beneficial effects. The brain tells the adrenal glands to stop producing adrenalin, and it tells the pituitary gland and the hypothalamus to begin secreting endorphins. The two effects add together: the reduction in adrenalin makes you relax, and the increase in endorphins makes you happy. Overall, in following the rhythm set by the breath, the heart triggers a cascade of effects that lead to general relaxation.

Here is a breathing exercise that has an amazing impact on the heart rate. It also has an effect on both the endocrine and immune systems, and it gets your heart to resonate with your breathing.

When the breathing cycle settles down to about five seconds to breathe in and five seconds to breathe out, the heart naturally adopts this rhythm for its own accelerations and decelerations. I can only encourage you to try this. You will find that the resonance happens by itself. Settle yourself in a comfortable armchair, close your eyes and let your breathing and heartbeat find their natural rhythms. In less than two minutes, they will be following the same rhythm. You will feel more and more relaxed. As well, you will find yourself thinking more clearly. This is because the brain waves in your two cerebral hemispheres will become synchronized.

At night, when you are in bed, lie on your back and begin this exercise again. Once you have synchronized your breathing and heart rates, you will fall into a delightful sleep.

Immune system

When your blood flows more rapidly because you exercise, the cells of your immune system are also quicker at doing their job—running into and destroying pathogenic agents. And since they will recognize these pathogenic agents, they can react even more quickly the next time they run into them.

Joints and ligaments

There are more than 60 joints in your body: in your fingers, toes, wrists, elbows, shoulders, vertebrae, hips, knees and ankles. To keep them mobile, you have to move regularly.

Lack of exercise is often the basic cause of arthritis and osteoarthritis. Similarly, the ligaments that join the various bones together need to move if they are to remain elastic. Setting some time aside for stretching while exercising is a smart way to keep your ligaments healthy.

The brain

Neurons also need to be oxygenated. Exercise is good for mental balance. Dr. Servan-Schreiber has clearly shown that exercise is more effective than Prozac at keeping you in a good mood.[2]

Studies have shown that NK (natural killer) cells made by white blood cells, the first line of defense against viruses or bacteria, are very sensitive to emotions. When you are stressed, "they tend to abate or to stop multiplying." On the other hand, we are told, "the better we feel, the more energetically they do their job."[3]

The best foods

The book The Instinct to Heal caused a stir in the field of health. Writing about the omega-3 revolution, Dr. Servan-Schreiber and his colleagues highlight the degree to which hospital medicine has forgotten the fundamental link between nutrition and health. It is only with the quite recent development of complementary medicine that this link has, once again, come into the limelight.

1. The HeartMath website at www.heartmath.com

2. David Servan-Schreiber, *The Instinct to Heal*, Chapter 10, Prozac or Puma?

3. Ibid., p. 148

Dr. Servan-Schreiber writes: "It is really astonishing that it took modern medicine 2,500 years to come back to this finding, an , be they Tibetan, Chinese, Ayurvedic, or Greco-Roman, stressed in their very first texts." As Hippocrates wrote, more than 2,400 years ago: "Let food be your medicine and medicine be your food."

Did you know that the cells of your body are born and die very frequently? In a single year, 98% of them disappear and are replaced! The lifespan of a bone cell? Three months. That of a liver cell? Six weeks. A skin cell? Four to six weeks. A cell from the inner lining of the stomach? Five days. With a lifespan of one year, brain cells live an astonishingly long time.

So where do we find the chemical elements needed to replace these millions of cells? In food, of course! Eating is the only way to replace our dead cells. We may think that we eat to please our palates, our eyes, or our stomachs, but really, we eat not to die. More than 100,000 persons on this planet die of hunger every day. These 100,000 people could not find the food their cells needed to replicate themselves before dying.

> Eating is the only way to replace our dead cells.

Why take care of my skin?

> Caring for your skin is also a way of taking care of your internal image.

There is a lovely expression in my language in which we describe people as "comfortable in their skins," or "uncomfortable in their skins," to indicate whether or not they feel good about themselves. These types of expressions clearly show how strong the links are between our external appearance and our inner life. Caring for your skin is not just a way of paying attention to your physical appearance. It is also a way of taking care of your internal image.

Moreover, our face and body have an impact on others. We are very sensitive to the body language of people we meet. We can easily read their interest, desire, indifference, or discomfort.

Without needing to put it into words, people communicate messages such as, "Hey, you look great!" or "You don't seem all that well." They can tell how well we are from the look of our skin, whether it is dull or shiny. Extremities of the body such as nails and hair also play a role in making you look either young or old.

So, in taking care of your skin you are also taking care of your relations with others. A beautiful skin, therefore, is rightly seen as a sign of youth, because it is the very essence of youthfulness!

With an area of some 22 square feet, the skin is the largest organ of the body. Its role is to protect us from the environment.

It has organs for eliminating wastes: the sudoriferous (or sweat) glands. It also has organs to maintain its own good health: the sebaceous glands. Dead cells and debris from microorganisms and cells flake off from the skin and are thus eliminated. The skin and its pores need to be clean for sweat to reach the surface. Basic skincare means keeping the pores free of dust, pollutants, and of excess sebum excretion and dead cells.

For those born with a genetic predisposition to be *red ovals* or *white circles*, it is a simple matter to preserve the skin's functions of protecting, maintaining and eliminating wastes. All it takes is a little water and some cleansing products. Aside from redness and sensitivity, *red ovals* and *white circles* do not really have skin problems. But that redness as well as their delicate skin, however, can lead to other problems. In particular, they have less protection from UV and a possible predisposition to melanoma.

Imbalances and a whole series of disorders appear more readily in *green squares* and *yellow rectangles*. Cleansing regularly is not enough for these types. They have to help their skin with anti-wrinkle products, or with products that stimulate the blood circulation and the oxygenation of their skin.

An imbalanced *green square* or *yellow rectangle* may develop eczema plaques or eruptions of acne due to an excess of sebum or, inversely, may develop a very dry, alipidic skin. Such types can also have hydration problems and may be at risk of developing expression wrinkles and appearing tired and grayish. Their skin might look older than it really is. But today we know that if you look after your skin properly, you can take off 10 to 15 years of fatigue and premature aging.

Today we know that if you look after your skin properly, you can take off 10 to 15 years of fatigue and premature aging.

Interpersonal relations and aging

Several studies have tried to identify what it is that makes people happy.

Mihaly Csikszentmihalyi, a psychologist of Hungarian origin and a professor at the University of Chicago, has been interested all his life in what brings happiness.

He characterizes happiness as being in the state of "flow." This is the state in which we are so involved in an activity that we become oblivious to our worries, to the passage of time and even to our own identities. We become one with what we are doing. We stop thinking about either the past or the future. We are caught

Skincare for all types

Here are some tips:

- In the evening, begin by cleaning the skin well. Before showering, remove your makeup or lift off dirt with a non-comedogenic cleansing milk which does not block pores. By doing this, you will not only remove your makeup, but also any impurities that have accumulated during the day.
- Whether it comes from the shower or from the tap, water has a pH of around 7. This is much too alkaline for the skin. Though it may seem like a paradoxical, it is true: city water is the worst water of all for the skin and ages it prematurely! To re-establish the pH of your skin, always use a solution or lotion with an acidic pH.
- A gentle foaming cleanser or gel is fine for cleaning your body. Use a foamy, bacteriostatic cleanser.
- When you have finished showering and dried your skin, use a contour gel around the eyes. Finish with a treatment cream for the face, chosen according to your type.
- In the morning, apply a small amount of moisturizing cream. You may then add a gel that fights the appearance of bags under the eyes, wrinkles or dark circles around the eyes. If you have to go outdoors, apply a sunscreen that is rated at least 15 SPF, which will protect you from both UVA and UVB and that contains antioxidants.
- If you wish to apply makeup, select a foundation with sunscreen in it.

Your skin may need special care as well as this basic maintenance. It may lack elasticity, it may be too oily, too dry, or too sensitive, or it may have an excess of capillaries or wrinkles. You may notice brown marks or acne. Later in this book, we will discuss the special products that exist for treating each of these kinds of imbalance. You will find more detail in the sections on skincare for each of the four body types. In general, the pH of healthy skin varies between 5.2 and 5.8; the ideal pH for skin is 5.5. It is important to preserve the skin's hydrolipic film through exfoliation and by using moisturizers and trace elements to maintain skin health and allow it to assume its protective role.

Preventive maintenance

Here are two simple rules for looking after your skin on a daily basis:

- ❖ Work out a simple routine. If you do not keep it simple, you will probably give it up after a few days.
- ❖ It is not the quantity of skincare products you use that will make the difference, but the quality. Choose products based on natural active ingredients and select those with proven results.

up intensely in the present. We float on a little cloud, simultaneously aware, active and relaxed, effortlessly coordinating our gestures. We do what we do automatically, as if by magic. This is happiness: action that flows without stress, obstacles, or turbulence.

Similarly, Dr. Servan-Schreiber has identified two factors that are always present in the lives of happy people. He writes: "Studies of people who are happier about their lives than others systematically point to two factors. Such people have close, stable, emotional relationships with others, and they are involved in their community."[4]

When I asked myself what to include in the cure for anti-aging that I was developing, it was obvious to me that it was necessary to include physical exercise and nutrition, as well as techniques for caring for the skin. But I also wanted to include interpersonal relations. This provides the balance. These aspects considered as a whole constitute the objective of the cure.

Physical exercise and nutrition, techniques for caring for your skin, and interpersonal relations provide a balance.

I have met many people who look worn out, with premature wrinkles and gray, lifeless complexions, who tell me about the tensions of their life at home or at work. I knew I had to address this: I had to add the dimension of emotions and relations to the three other dimensions in my method in order for the anti-aging cure to be complete.

When I learned about the experimental studies of the HeartMath[1] Institute, I realized that the conclusions I had reached from my professional experience with over 5,000 clients were actually the same facts that these studies now proved beyond a

4. David Servan-Schreiber, *The Instinct to Heal*, Chapter 14, p. 211.

When you feel comfortable with the people around you, the effects are physiological. You are in balance.

doubt. When you feel comfortable with the people around you, the effects are physiological. You are in balance. Your body works well, much better than when you live with stress and worry. You feel both clearer in your thoughts and surer in your affections. Your cells regain their suppleness and adaptability—the two key characteristics of youth.

There is no question that when we influence our physiology through breathing, exercise, skincare and nutrition, our feelings about ourselves and those around us change. And the way others feel about us changes as well.

Western medicine is beginning to realize that interpersonal relations are in themselves intervention tools. This realization began in the first specialized clinics for treating pain, which were created in the United States at the beginning of the 1960s. The idea has spread slowly, to many but not to all of the healthcare professions. As Dr. Servan-Schreiber writes with a hint of frustration: "The idea that a loving relationship is in itself a physiological remedy, comparable to taking medication, rests on sound scientific ground—but it simply has not yet taken hold in the medical establishment."[6]

I began observing the interpersonal relations of my clients, in the context of their lives as couples, workers and family members. These relations developed differently, depending on whether they were *red ovals*, *green squares*, *yellow rectangles*, or *white circles*. I noticed that they did not try to get me to solve problems for them. I also noticed that they always had more resources than they thought they had. They simply needed me to point them in the right direction, to supply them with the tools that had already been shown to work for people like them.

5. Doc Childre, *One minute stress management.*

Red Ovals

Physical exercise

What *red ovals* have a tendency to do

Because they are feckless or impulsive, *red ovals* tend to overexercise. During a period of imbalance, they will be also be inclined to overexert themselves. For example, they will pedal too quickly for their tendons, or lift weights that are too heavy for their muscles. Similarly, they will ignore warm-up periods, as if they are just in too much of a rush to get sweaty and to lose their excess weight right away.

Because they have low self-esteem and are easily influenced, they will be drawn to whatever exercise is in fashion, such as Pilates, tai chi, kickboxing, or the latest diet everyone is talking about. They will happily follow the advice of a professional, but will not keep it up for long.

What they should not do

Avoid exercises that you do standing up. It would be preferable to do your cardio exercises on a bicycle, for example. Do other exercises while stretched out on the floor. Wear compression stockings if you are a woman, and tension bandages if you are a man (or apply a complex of essential oils). Put them on while you are still lying on the floor.

What they should do

In general, the objective of physical exercise for *red ovals* is to correct, at an early stage, the imbalances to which they are subject. *Red ovals* have to fight against their propensity to vasodilatation in the arteries and veins.

Red ovals have to fight against their propensity to vasodilatation in the arteries and veins.

Cardiovascular exercise

❖ Unless you are quite fit, twenty minutes per day is all it takes! Excessiveness in doing cardiovascular exercise is not good for *red ovals*. If you have a treadmill or a stationary bicycle, exercise at a pace that is brisk but not punishing. Do not set a slope on the treadmill. Your heart should speed up, but not too much. Keep your heart rate below 130 beats per minute. A brisk bike ride could well substitute for a session on the treadmill.

❖ Afterwards, lie on your back with your legs straight and against a wall and rest without moving for five minutes. This will help the blood flow back towards your heart.

❖ It would be a good idea to put a large book under the foot of your mattress and leave it there. It is good for you to keep your feet a little higher than the rest of your body during the night.

Building muscle and stretching

Three times a week, 20 minutes in total for each series.

❖ *Red ovals* usually have poorly developed abdominal muscles. Begin on the floor, lying on your back. First, do scissors with your legs to bring the blood back to your heart. Do a first series of 12 scissors, take a break, then do a second series.

❖ Rotate all the joints (articulations). Relax your muscles while rotating: relax your neck, your jaws, your arms, etc. Rotate to the right, to the left, to the front, then behind and to each side.

❖ Lift your legs. Lower them and, without touching the floor, lift them again. Repeat 12 times. Take a break and then begin another series of 12 leg lifts.

❖ Finish with sit-ups. Remember to place your hands behind your head and to spread your elbows far apart. This opens up your chest and encourages deep breathing. Do a series of 12; take a break, then start again.

❖ If you are living through a stressful time, try to find out where your muscles are tightest. For most people, it is usually in the neck and back.

❖ To stretch yourself still more, hang from a bar with your hands apart. Lift yourself up a little using the strength of your arms and then relax. Lift again, relax. What counts is not the number of times you lift yourself, but the degree to which you relax completely between lifts. Next, with your hands farther apart, begin the lifts again, followed by stretches using your own body weight. This will work your shoulders and release tension from your neck right down to the bottom of your back.

❖ Given your predisposition to flushing, do not overdo the exercises. Leave 48 hours between muscle-building workouts.

Nutrition

What *red ovals* have a tendency to do

Every *red oval* has a sweet tooth. When *red ovals* go to a restaurant they load up at the buffet and always return two or three times to the desserts! Not only do they love sugar, but they also have trouble resisting temptation. It is very hard for them to say "No, thank you," to chocolate cakes or cheesecakes, or to resist fruit pies covered with thick syrup or a mouthwateringly colorful coulis! It is worse when the person beside them has second and third helpings of something really delicious. For *red ovals*, the tendency to eat sweets is reinforced by the tendency to do what others do.

What they should not do

For the sake of your health, learn to identify and avoid what is not good for you. Let others make their choices: they are, by nature, different from you. If they know their type, their natural diet could be radically different from yours. If they have already learned to say "Yes" to what is good for them and "No" to what is bad for them, then you can let yourself be influenced by their search for balance, but not by their choices!

Would you like some good advice? Cut out half of all foods such as pasta, cheese, or bread that contain yeast, sugar, or any of the other substances that digestion converts into sugars or toxins. During my career I have often recommended Dr. William Crook's book, *The Yeast Connection,* which documents the role of yeast and its impact on health.

If you have high blood pressure, you are going to see a clear difference within a few weeks. If you have asthma, this simple decision is going to lessen considerably the intensity and the frequency of your attacks. If you are a woman who tends to have vaginal discharge, it will not only decrease, but you will also feel a boost of fresh energy.

Avoid foods that have been sitting for hours on the table: they oxidize quickly when exposed to daylight and air. Instead, eat what has been freshly harvested or freshly prepared for you. Avoid cheeses that have exposed to the air for a long time or that contain molds, because they will make you feel bloated.

Cut out half of all foods such as pasta, cheese, or bread that contain yeast, sugar, or any of the other substances that digestion converts into sugars or toxins.

Similarly, avoid products that stimulate the circulation such as spices, caffeine, alcohol and cigarettes. They dilate the blood vessels and raise your blood pressure. Some of your capillaries may burst, causing red flushes that will not go away unless you have them removed; you should avoid anything that might aggravate your natural tendency towards vasodilatation.

You should also avoid eating anything that generates acidity in the stomach: fried foods, processed foods, carbonated drinks, cold meats, jams and deli foods.

Salt is not good for you because it causes the tissues to retain water, and you already have a tendency towards developing edema.

What they should do

The most important thing is to drink lots of water. Take your first glass as soon as you get up in the morning. Drink several glasses during the day with a little lemon zest. Eat colored vegetables: broccoli; carrots; green, yellow, red or orange peppers; green or yellow beans, etc.

Drink a soothing herbal tea such as chamomile, millepertuis (St. John's wort) or hawthorn to ease your tendency towards becoming flushed. Do not drink too much, of course, or you will just fall asleep!

Skincare

What *red ovals* have a tendency to do

Red ovals have extremely sensitive skin, with a very thin epidermis. Genetically, *red ovals* are predisposed to flushing, which may become aggravated over time and turn into rosacea and its various stages such as couperose (telangiectasia). *Red ovals* love perfumes, essences, creams and bath soaps and they will put almost anything on their skin. They also have a taste for novelty and want to try whatever gadgets are new and fashionable.

What they should not do

Above all, *red ovals* should avoid products that irritate and destroy the hydrolipic barrier, such as soaps (generally alkaline) or creams with alpha hydroxy acids (AHA), or that contain lactic, citric, malic, or glycolic acids in concentrations of 10% or more. They should not use any product with a low pH (3.5 or less). Such products are not good for this kind of skin.

Red ovals should avoid microdermabrasion, micro-current treatments, and lifting devices that stimulate blood circulation.

They should avoid hot baths and saunas. If you are a *red oval* and just cannot do without such a treatment, you should at least limit its duration because you are going to perspire so much that your skin will become dehydrated, leaving it prone to becoming dry and developing a mineral imbalance.

One of the advantages of being a *red oval* is that you do not need anti-wrinkle cream. Everything is a question of balance. For your eyelids, use a light gel but never use a cream. Creams always have an oil base, which causes the delicate skin of the eyelids to swell.

Avoid vitamin A acid, which may sometimes be prescribed for you, because it has exfoliant properties. Since your epidermis is naturally very thin, it is important not to make it even thinner.

Use a bacteriostatic cleanser if you have acne rosacea. Avoid antibacterial cleansers, even if they are recommended to you, because they destroy the enzymes that preserve your hydrolipic barrier.

One of the advantages of being a *red oval* is that you do not need anti-wrinkle cream.

What they should do

Red ovals should put on a sunscreen with high sun-protection factor (preferably an SPF of 30 or more) every day. Make sure that your sunscreen protects against both UVA (with physical filters) and UVB, and that it contains antioxidants.

Your goals, when visiting a skincare professional, should always be to:

- ❖ Protect your arterial capillaries from vasodilation by using anti-flushing products such as bioflavonoids, rosehips, or rutin;
- ❖ Mineralize your skin by taking an oligo-element complex such as silicon or magnesium;
- ❖ Improve venous and lymphatic drainage through massage;
- ❖ Avoid all exfoliating or circulation-stimulating procedures, such as chemical peelings or micro-currents, unless they are very gentle and non-irritating;

❖ Avoid any extraction process for comedons (blackheads).

Since you are attracted by the newest technology, you will be tempted to try the latest, most fashionable equipment. Do not give in to this temptation. First, find out if the tempting new process will stimulate your blood circulation (this is to be avoided), so that you can make a decision independent of any recommendations you have received. Above all, think of yourself and your true nature!

Interpersonal communications

Within the couple

A *red oval* should ideally pair up with a *green square*. The two complement each other very well. The *red oval* contributes insouciance, good humor and love of life, while the *green square* contributes the ability to see things clearly and to pay attention to details. While the *red oval* impulsively spends, the *green square* compulsively calculates. The *red oval* is the cricket that sings all summer long, while the *green square* is the ant busily storing provisions for winter.

But not all *red ovals* find their *green squares*. What is in store for you? You are probably going to succumb to various temptations, and this is going to create tension with your partner.

Imagine, for instance, that you run into friends. Happy to see them, you invite them home for dinner without first checking with your partner. *Red oval* that you are, you have made a spontaneous, friendly gesture. You like having the house full of life. But you have not thought about your partner, who hates being disturbed and having to improvise. It is not that your partner dislikes your friends; it is just that he or she does not feel ready to receive them, does not like being faced with a done deal, and anyway there is nothing in the fridge to make something decent for guests. When you planned your pleasant surprise and surprised your partner with, "Guess who's coming to dinner?" you expected a smile. But unfortunately, instead of joy, you have only generated anxiety. As a *green square*, your partner would have appreciated being part of the decision-making process.

Here is another example. You spot the newest DVD player in a store window. It is the very model you noticed and admired at a friend's the previous evening. Even though you cannot really afford it, you go into the store and buy it. Consequence? Your

Exercise 5.

All curves: chest, waist, buttocks

Now that you have become a better observer, let's change how we observe. Instead of randomly observing individuals and figuring out their body types from their characteristics, we will do the opposite. We will find types with strongly marked characteristics and observe them in detail.

Position yourself in a place from which you can observe dozens of people. Note that quantity is essential for this exercise. There is no use trying it if you can only observe five or six subjects.

We are looking for several *red ovals*.

❖ Following the usual sequence, first find people who belong in the ample family.

❖ From these amples, pick those with reddish-pink skin, rounded muscles and generous curves. In other words, identify those who are easily classed as *red ovals*.

❖ Review the characteristics of the type, point by point, for each of the subjects thus clearly identified.

• Color palette
• Forms and proportions of the face
• Forms and proportions of the body
• Distinctive signs

Note those aspects that match the classification of *red oval* and those that point to another type. Pay particular attention to the chest, buttocks and breasts. Gentlemen, if you do not want to get slapped in the face you should make your observations discreetly, or wear dark glasses!

Duration: 30 minutes

partner is mad at you for not having being consulted. They had already budgeted for the purchase of some other piece of equipment that month.

Or consider the following scenario. Because your partner makes a simple mistake, you get angry and use harsh, excessive, unfair words. Ten minutes later, you have forgotten the incident, but your partner is still trying to figure out why you blew up, smarting from the sting of your hurtful, bitter words. You should be aware that you speak freely and have a quick temper, and can wound others without even knowing it.

You speak freely and have a quick temper, and can wound others without even knowing it.

So, what should you do about your impulsive temperament? Simply ask yourself why you act the way you do.

So, what should you do about your impulsive temperament? Simply ask yourself why you act the way you do.

Let me make a suggestion. You always seem to be reacting to something. Whether yielding to the joy of conviviality, impulsively shopping, or losing your temper, it seems that it is always your environment that determines your actions. You give the impression that you never say no, but rather simply react to some action or respond to some stimulus. It is as if you are missing some filter, as if you never step back for a moment to weigh the pros and cons of a proposed action.

You cannot change your nature, of course, but you can at least ask why you are always creating the kinds of situations that your partner finds difficult. True, you do not mean any harm; in fact, you love your partner more than anything in the world, and you know very well that you are essential for his or her happiness.

In fact, you are always looking for approval from your partner. But the things you do upset your partner, because you allow him or her so little time or space. So try to ask yourself the question: What is the reason for this behavior?

I am suggesting that you behave like this to others because you allow yourself so little time or space! You do not even allow yourself time to check your own decisions. In fact, they are not really decisions, just impetuous reactions. You are looking for approval in the eyes of your partner without having taken the time to find out whether you yourself approve of what you have just done!

Once you have reviewed all the reasons why you act the way you do, take note of them, but do not judge or blame yourself. Just be aware of these reasons and of the fact that they can influence your future conduct. Think of them as being part of you, no more, no less. You should not be trying to change your nature, but to realize its full potential. So carefully examine what you like best about your partner. You will discover how to keep your partner content, at the same time as you learn to thoroughly appreciate your own nature. For a couple, happiness lies in mutual balance and self-realization.

Here is another tip that might help. Stop comparing yourself and your partner with other couples. Do not always look elsewhere. You have heard people say unflattering things about your partner? Do not listen to them. You are too easily influenced. Instead, look at your partner's qualities. Think about the person who so pleased you when you first met. Surround yourself with people who find your partner charming.

Treat your partner generously, in ways that will reinforce the qualities that made you fall in love in the first place. Can you cook and choose fine wines? Then invite your friends over as often as you like, as long as you do the cooking. Prepare meals for your partner as you do for your friends. Do you have a good eye for comfort and decoration? Do you know how to arrange colors, fabrics and textures? Then why not redecorate a room in your home, with both you and your partner making the decisions? Are you good at planning trips? Then plan a trip that combines both relaxation and culture, with visits, lazy times, fine dining and physical activities. Surprise your partner on his or her birthday with your wonderful plan. If the trip is well thought out and carefully planned, he or she will not only be really surprised but really enthusiastic, and your beautiful surprise will not be spoiled by the necessity of sticking to a budget!

I could go on listing examples of what do to, but you get the idea; to succeed as a couple, think about actions that compensate for what your partner has too much or too little of and, at the same time, that suit your real nature. Learn to curb your impulses, and, as long as you do something that balances your partner's nature and realizes yours (and vice versa), you are going in the right direction. Remember, it is not always green on the other side...

At work

You like work that requires you to look after clients' needs. You would enjoy being a salesperson, for instance, or perhaps a decorator, travel agent, consultant, hairdresser, or caterer. You are comfortable with new technology, so you would be good with multimedia, state-of-the-art machinery, or cars. Women *red ovals* are drawn to jobs in which they can offer advice on clothing, skincare, diet and decoration. *Red ovals* love change, are very creative and are equally attracted to the arts, singing, performance and music.

The main problem for *red ovals* is their lack of self-confidence at work, despite the fact that they always bring good cheer to their teams. What their colleagues particularly appreciate is that *red ovals* are always good humored and always have a story to tell. But *red ovals* do not see themselves as others do.

So what can be done? The answer, in fact, is easy: just cultivate your good qualities. You were hired because of these qualities. Continue being a warm presence at meetings. Keep the wheels turning. Project a good mood when talking to clients on the phone. You are likeable. Whatever you do, do not change that. Your smile and energy are of great value. You need some way to measure the value of your work. You are like the cricket, who sings and gives generously, without ever measuring the results. You find the very idea of such measurements horrifying. But without any idea of how effective you are, you just have no way of knowing the value of your work. And since you have a rather negative image of yourself, you think that your work does not count for much!

Yet, in the end, you should realize that in not measuring anything, in not being aware of the real contribution that you make to the company, you are actually harming yourself. You are losing the chance of knowing what you are worth. Your horror of measurement is working against you. Yet now is probably the time to be aware that, as the saying goes, time is money. So calculate expenses, think about profit instead of sales, and start to measure, measure, and measure.

I guarantee you that you will come to like what you learn about yourself and your contributions at work. You will see that the gratitude you are always looking for will just come, by itself. In time, you will not even need it. It will be nice to have, but no more than that. It will just confirm what you already know. It will be based on what you really do contribute at work.

In concrete terms, you should begin every day by saying to yourself: "Today, I'm going to stop hiding from my boss. Instead, I'm going to ask how I can best measure my results." Your boss will be happy to see that you are trying to evaluate yourself against the standards and expectations of the company, to know that you are taking care of your own image, and that the goals of the company are well understood.

In the end, what is the most important thing for a business? It is not the opinion your colleagues have of you. It is whatever sells, whatever gets stock out of the warehouse, whatever adds value to the company's products—and what you do that has an influence on all that!

So give yourself the means to measure the value of what you contribute. Once your value has been established in terms that your business recognizes, the problem of appreciation for your work is over. All that remains is for you to make the little extra effort to acknowledge the numbers and to acknowledge that, when it comes to work, a salesperson is worth what he or she sells.

You will finally have the pleasure of knowing your own worth, without question or doubt; you will no longer be angling for encouraging little pats on the back. In conclusion, then, just be confident that your boss appreciates your work and stop worrying that you are going to fail or be fired.

When it comes to relations with your family, however, what you have to do is quite different.

Within the family

Have you noticed that you never talk about yourself to your family? Yes, of course, you make them laugh, you tell them stories, you play with them and you love them, there is no doubt about that. You are trying to give them what you felt you were not lucky enough to receive.

Your children love you unconditionally. You are a hero to them. It would be a good idea, though, to lower your voice when talking to them and to be careful about not being too impulsive in making decisions that concern them.

Do they know that their hero is self-doubting and sometimes only pretends to be happy? No, they do not really know this, but they do suspect it a little, for kids have extraordinary intuition and ears that are always finely tuned!

As you yourself know only too well. When you were a kid, you were always trying to figure out what your parents really felt about you. Yet what you are doing now is trying to hide who you really are deep down from your own kids. Why? Quite simply because you want to be a superhero.

It is ironic, isn't it? You offer them the love you felt you never got, but you hide the reason why you want them to have it all.

You want to be a superhero.

You do not want to let them down. You think that they would be really disappointed if they were to discover the real you. So what do you do? You keep all your doubts, your limits and what you do not like about yourself well hidden.

But have you ever thought about what your children think of you? For them, you are the best mom or dad in the world. They have no idea that you feel you were under-appreciated as a child. By omission, you are telling a lie. There is no need to hide your feelings about yourself from them. They have an accurate idea of your worth. Who could be in a better position to appreciate how good you are as a mother or a father? And they are ready to tell you. If you ask them, they can tell you exactly what you are worth; but as long as you carefully avoid the subject, they will not talk.

So allow me to give you some good advice. Forget your pride and tell them that you love them. Tell them how much you wished you had been told this when you were their age. As everybody knows, self-confidence comes from knowing that you are loved. And then you can ask the following question. "Tell me, what do you think of this?" And why not give them a few compliments? You are going to make several people happy:

- You are going to make your kids and family feel good because you trust and respect their opinion.
- You are going to feel good yourself when you get in touch with what they are thinking.

Case study: *red oval*

Two meetings for a desperate *red oval!*

*I*n the San Francisco office of a well-known doctor, I had an appointment with a client who was utterly desperate. She had tried everything to get rid of her cellulite: 26 endermology sessions, a strict diet, algae wraps, essential oils, naturopathy, massotherapy and even liposuction. Nothing worked. Then she saw a newspaper advertisement about my upcoming clinic, and, though she was skeptical and disillusioned, she said to herself, "I'll try just one more time, but this is really going to be the last time."

Well-dressed, in her early 40s, alert and educated, a lawyer, this woman was a *red oval*.

Linda listed her symptoms for me: she had numbness in her legs and, at night, cramps that were painful enough to wake her. She also had cellulite that she had tried to treat, but had not obtained satisfactory results.

I asked her to undress for an examination. There were several signs of problems with her venous and lymphatic circulation. Her upper thighs were very edematous. The vessels of the great saphenous vein were dilated and distinctly visible. It is easy to notice venous insufficiency and imbalance in lymphatic circulation; the hydric cellulite is clearly evident.

I suggested that she consult a doctor, because I suspected she had a venous problem, and that she have a duplex ultrasound scan to check the circulation in her lower limbs.

I then explained to her why, given these problems, the treatments she had previously tried could not work well on her:

- her venous insufficiency meant that toxins were being recirculated;
- algae wrappings could only aggravate her condition by worsening her circulatory problems;
- liposuction did remove fat, but in doing so destroyed numerous vessels damaging lymphatic channels, blocked free drainage.

By the flushing in her face, I could see right away that she had symptoms of rosacea. In the conversation that followed, Linda told me that her skin felt sore as soon as she stepped outdoors. To avoid wrinkles, she told me that she used a cream with an alpha hydroxy acid (AHA) base, and that it stung her face as soon as she applied it.

It is an obvious error for a person of her type to use such creams: they have an exfoliating action when the pH is low. Linda did not need exfoliation. As a *red oval*, her skin was thin and was genetically predisposed to hypersensitivity and to flushing.

The solution for her was to protect her arterial capillaries. She also needed a vasoconstricting serum for her venous capillaries, a vasodilating serum for the lymphatic capillaries, a protective cream to balance and hydrate her skin and, finally, a sunscreen to avoid further damage to her face.

Anti-aging cure for Linda

- Before getting out of bed, apply to your legs a complex of essential oils in spray form with a high concentration of horse chestnut and arnica to promote vasoconstriction of the venous capillaries;

- Put on a custom-made medical compression stocking. Take a shower or bath in the evening;
- Before getting out of bed, do cardiovascular exercises. Lie on your side, lift your legs in the air and make pedaling motions for 20 minutes every day;
- After exercising, clean your skin with a cleanser for sensitive skin and use an acidic pH toner;
- Before going out, put on a sunscreen with SPF of 30 or greater, UVA and UVB protection and anti-oxidants;
- During the day, do 10 minutes of cycling. Drink one glass of water for every 10 pounds (4.5 kg) of weight (12 glasses if you weigh 120 pounds (55 kg), for example);
- At the midday and evening meals take a food supplement of 350 mg of magnesium and calcium combined, a 500 mg supplement of bioflavonoids and vitamin C to improve circulation, a multivitamin complex and 100 mg of alpha-lipoic acid. Eat three garlic cloves or the equivalent in capsules every day;
- In the evening, take a shower or a lukewarm bath with vasoconstricting essential oils such as wild mint, cypress, or sandalwood;
- Visit a clinic three times a week during five weeks for a series of 15 20-minute pressotherapy treatments. Use compression stockings to reduce venous insufficiency and lymphatic edema and to improve cellulite;
- Ideally, if possible, take two sessions of lymphatic drainage massage per week during two weeks.

Three weeks later, Linda returned for a second appointment. The redness in her face had already considerably diminished. When she went outside her skin hurt much less.

Two months later Linda sent me a lovely thank-you letter. "Manon," she wrote, "you were the only specialist to diagnose the real problem and to suggest the right kind of treatment. In fact, the duplex ultrasound scan confirmed your hypothesis of a venous problem." Her cramps and numbness had now gone away, she added. Her skin was smooth once again, and the appearance of her legs improved so that she could wear shorts and a swimsuit.

Games

1. Amples or angulars?

Identify each class to which these statements apply:

1.	I have thin skin	
2.	My nervous system is particularly active.	
3.	I tend to be generously curved.	
4.	I am often cold, or have cold extremities.	
5.	I have a poor circulatory system.	
6.	My muscles are either well-defined, or long and delicate.	
7.	My jaw is rather round.	
8.	My skin tone ranges from yellow to green.	
9.	My epidermis is thick.	
10.	Most models and dancers belong to this class.	

2. What type?

Identify the first type that comes to mind when you hear these sentences:

1.	My hands and feet are always cold.	
2.	I feel weak unless I have several snacks during the day. Fortunately, I never gain an ounce.	
3.	My skin turns red after a couple of seconds in the sun and, moreover, I feel warm all the time.	
4.	In the morning, my legs feel heavy and sometimes they hurt. Even in the summer I never leave the house without a jacket because I always feel chilly.	
5.	Even in the summer I never leave the house without a jacket because I always feel chilly.	
6.	I sweat a lot.	
7.	When I go to the gym my muscles quickly become sculpted and I look like an athlete.	
8.	I sweat when I eat spicy food.	

Green Squares

Physical exercise

What *green squares* have tendency to do

By nature, *green squares* are extremists. When it comes to exercise, they either do a lot or none at all. One thing is for sure: when *green squares* exercise, they do not take half measures. They will arrange it so that there is a bit of an exclusive side to their training sessions. They will want personal trainers, or specially adapted machines. Otherwise, when a *green square* is alone in the gym, he or she will pretend to know everything. *Green squares* are the kind of people who will exercise in exchange for some reward: for their health, for AIR MILES®, for merit points, or for their own physical comfort.

What they should not do

There are no exercises that *green squares* should avoid. They are naturally talented and can do anything. They should resist the tendency to be excessive, however; to avoid developing stretch marks, they should not do weight lifting and increase weights too rapidly, or let exercise sessions last too long.

Green squares should also resist their tendency to think constantly about things such as work, multiple projects and their upcoming engagements.

What they should do

What makes *green squares* age is uncontrolled stress. Rebalancing their nervous systems, giving a greater role to the sympathetic system, can keep them looking young. Their best choice, then, is to learn how to relax and do nothing and how to sleep well.

Green squares need a good reason to exercise[6]. Often this reason is to be able to do something else at the same time: to watch the news while riding a stationary bicycle, for example, or to get real-time data about their cardiac and respiratory rhythms, the

> What makes *green squares* age is uncontrolled stress.

6. David Servan-Schreiber, *The Instinct to Heal*, Chapter 11, p. 173.

number of paces made, distance covered, or to win air miles or cash, etc.

Green squares tend to think that they work best under stress, and they do not want to feel that they are wasting time by exercising.

Some of the recommended ways for *green squares* to relax include listening to music, taking a bath, reading, or being read to. Anything that can distract them from the world outside and help them discover the world inside will help them. *Green squares* have such a strong inclination to be at the mercy of the pressures of the outside world and, in turn, to put pressure on those around them, that they can forget to have an inner life.

They should be doing activities such as yoga, meditation and massage, which will reduce their anxiety, allow them to clear their mind, and help teach them that the body exists not only to crank out work but also to rest and relax. Massages of the neck, especially the nape, and of the scalp are highly recommended to help *green squares* relax.

Green squares have such a strong inclination to be at the mercy of the pressures of the outside world and, in turn, to put pressure on those around them, that they can forget to have an inner life.

A self-massage for *green squares*

Are you a stressed out *green square*? Yes? Well then, here is good news: you can do yourself a world of good just with your ten fingers. Raise your arms and place your hands on each side of your neck, at the base of your nape. Synchronize your breathing with your heart rate: breathe in for five seconds, hold for five seconds, breathe out for five seconds. With the tips of your fingers, press in towards the central part of your neck. Press, then release. Press, then release. Repeat a dozen times. Take the time to sense the effect. Is your skin warmer? Do you feel some tingling? Let your head fall forward, then raise it and begin massaging with your fingertips again. It is normal to find yourself swallowing, as toxic wastes are being released. Does your body feel more alive now?

Suppleness

In *green squares*, the muscles around the kidneys, at the level of lumbar vertebrae L1 and L2, are often stiff. *Green squares* are prone to back pain, particularly in the lumbar region. What they do not know is that they often suffer from problems of toxin build up. They feel the weakness in their intestines and in their lower back.

Here are two exercises that *green squares* can do to help relax the lower back. The first is really simple. The second is more of a challenge.

Green squares are prone to back pain, particularly in the lumbar region.

Unrolling the back

❖ Stand with your feet shoulder-width apart, with your arms hanging down by your sides. Slowly bend your neck so that your head hangs down in front, stretching your neck with its weight. Relax your shoulders and let your arms hang down, heavy and relaxed. Then bend forwards, very slowly, letting your head and then your arms approach the floor. All your back will be stretched, one vertebra at a time. Let your natural elasticity determine how far you bend over. It is fine if your hands do not go any lower than your knees. Note how far you bend over and compare with how you do next time. If your hands can reach as low as your calves or your ankles, that is even better. If your back is sufficiently supple that you can put your hands palm down on the ground, that is perfect. Never force anything. The goal is to explore how supple your back is. It would be worthwhile repeating this every day.

❖ While doing this exercise, pay attention to what happens when you inhale and when you exhale. You will have a tendency to lift a little when inhaling. On every exhalation, your hands will be able to go down a little lower. Just make a note of what is happening and do not force your breathing.

❖ When you feel that your hands can go no lower, lift yourself slowly back to the starting position. Repeat the exercise. The whole sequence should last no more than five minutes. You might think you do not have time for exercise, but you cannot tell me you do not have five minutes to spare!

Progressive rotation of the lower back

❖ Lie on your back on the floor, with your arms stretcheout like a cross. Turn your head so you can see your left hand. Relax your neck completely. Lift your left knee above your hip and then, while still looking at your left hand, gently lower your left knee to the ground on your right side. You will soon feel a rotating stretch in your back.

❖ Do not force it. Stop if you feel any pain. Let the weight of your left leg apply the rotating stretch to your back. If you can touch the ground with your left foot, that is fine, but that is not the goal. The goal is to see how far you can reach and to notice that your foot gets closer to the ground each time you try the exercise. Make sure that both your shoulders stay touching the ground.

❖ Place your left leg back where it began and now do the same thing on the other side. Look at your right hand, letting your neck relax. Lift your right knee above your hip. Then, while continuing to look at your right hand, let your right knee drop on your left side, gently stretching your back. Observe how far you can go without exerting any force and stop at that point. Observe the effect of your breathing on the stretch. On breathing out, your right leg is lowered a little farther under its own weight. Do this exercise two times on each side.

Cardio

❖ Women should wear a sports bra when doing these exercises.

❖ Here is an exercise that will remind you of your childhood and increase your heart rate while you are having fun. The game is to make eight jumps forward, spending as little time as possible on the ground. It is like being in a sack race without a sack. If you do not have enough room in a corridor at home to take a sequence of eight jumps, then jump in a circle, turning a little to one side at each jump. It is not the distance you jump that counts, but the speed at which you jump. Take a break after each series of eight jumps. Repeat five times.

❖ To increase you heart rate still further, do the same exercise again but this time lift your knees as high as you can on each jump. Swing your arms forward every time you jump. You will find that you warm up quickly and your heart will jump with joy. If you have a device for taking your pulse, you will notice that it is above 100 beats per minute.

❖ *Green squares* love activities in which they get together with friends. A *green square* could easily sell his or her colleagues on the advantages of what is called spinning or group cycling. Nowadays, sports clubs have rooms in which a series of racing bicycles are placed in front of a screen. A trainer plays a film and, surprise, the speed at which you cycle matches the content of the film. Everybody accelerates when going down a hill and slows down going up a hill, when pedaling

Green squares have such a strong inclination to be at the mercy of the pressures of the outside world and, in turn, to put pressure on those around them, that they can forget to have an inner life.

becomes more difficult. It is like an interactive film, or an arcade video game, except that everything is arranged for the cyclists to pedal as a team, under the guidance of a trainer. With its competitive aspects, spinning is just the kind of activity that a *green square* would enjoy and do regularly.

Muscle building

- Here is an exercise that will strengthen your lower back. Adapt these instructions to the space you will use. For example, if you are exercising at home, use your bedroom and sit down on the floor at the foot of your bed. Stretch out on your back, lift your legs, and place them on the bed, with the insides of your knees on the end of the bed. Stretch out your arms on each side of your body.
- Lift your hips as high as you can, pushing up with your heels on the bed, supporting yourself with your arms on the floor.
- Then lower your hips to the floor. Raise and lower your hips like this 10 times in a row, then rest before doing another series. At the beginning of the exercise, it is just the leg muscles that are working, pushing against the bed. To lift your buttocks up even higher, you have to use the muscles of the lower back. Try to feel the moment when these muscles begin to work. In *green squares*, these muscles (the quadratus lumborum, gluteus maximus and iliopsoas) tend to be tight. It is a good idea to learn where they are located and to be able to tense and relax them independently.
- Here is an excellent exercise for *green squares* who go to the gym. Install light weights on a vertical pull-down apparatus. The goal is not to force, but to isolate the two groups known as the greater and smaller pectoral muscles and the trapezius muscle.
- Keep your breathing steady, in for five seconds, hold for five seconds, and out for five second. With arms outstretched, reach for the handles of the horizontal bar while breathing out, and slowly pull the bar down to the level of the nape of your neck.
- Keep your chest out while pulling the bar down.
- Then slowly let the bar rise, resisting the upward pull of the weights. Breathe in while the bar rises.

❖ Add muscle-building exercises with weights. Do not let a weight training session last more than 20 to 45 minutes, and do not do more than three sessions per week. Increase weights very gradually and work all your muscle groups, with 12 repetitions (two times) for each muscle group.

Nutrition

What *green squares* have a tendency to do

When *green squares* give into their inclinations, they eat salty foods such as chips, fries, pretzels, salami and smoked meat. In short, they prefer to take things with more than a grain of salt!

As well as such salty foods, they also like carbohydrates like pasta and potatoes, cream and cheeses such as mozzarella and Port-Salut that are at least 50% fat and bland in taste.

What is amazing is that *green squares* like to prepare food, but are somewhat indifferent to the pleasures of eating. They would be just as happy if they could nourish themselves simply by taking pills or injections.

What they should not do

Unfortunately, *green squares* should avoid the three things they most like: salt, carbohydrates and saturated fats.

They are drawn to saturated fats, but have trouble digesting them. Among women with cellulite, those who are *green squares* and who eat chips and pork have the most fibrous cellulite, which is the hardest to eliminate.

Salty foods make *green squares* salivate, but they would be better off getting their ration of iodine by eating seafood from time to time and in moderation. Salt aggravates their genetic predisposition to heart problems, diseases such as arteriosclerosis and strokes.

Carbonara pasta, with cream, salt, cheese and carbohydrates all together, is their favorite kind of dish. The fact that *green squares* have trouble digesting fatty cheeses makes them prone to get candida albicans and causes constipation.[7] Moreover, they have difficulty transforming the starch in pasta into sugar. When they

Unfortunately, *green squares* should avoid the three things they most like: salt, carbohydrates and saturated fats.

7. See *The Yeast Connection* by Dr. William G. Crook

give into their favorite temptation, they feel bloated, have gas, have headaches, or sleep poorly. Let's be even clearer. Their back pain is often linked to the fact that their colon is badly lubricated and unbalanced, and their constipation can be blamed on their difficulty digesting the yeasts in cheese and carbohydrates.

What they should do

Everybody, including *green squares*, needs fat. The important thing is not to stop eating fat, but to eat only good fats. *Green squares* can eat as much fat as they like as long as they eat the right kind: essential oils such as omega-3, omega-8, or omega–9 complexes, those found in borage, olive, or flax oil, or in salmon.

Green squares easily digest white meat (chicken, turkey, duck) and freshwater fish or fish from northern oceans. They can eat such meat or fish grilled on charcoal or in the oven, but they should not eat the skin.

To lubricate their colons and facilitate elimination, *green squares* need more fiber than do other types. Vegetables, either raw or steamed, are a convenient source of such fiber. Celery, cauliflower, broccoli, soy bean sprouts, radishes or watercress, sourdough bread and wheat germ (a source of vitamin E) all aid in regular and painless elimination. These vegetables could be prepared in a blender and consumed fresh.

Green squares who have real problems with digestion and constipation should add food supplements known to clean the liver to this fiber-rich food.

Colonic massage stimulates the peristaltic reflex and helps elimination. Recommended are gliding, kneading and vibratory massage strokes that first rise up, then go across, then descend down the colon in a clockwise motion.

Skincare

What *green squares* have a tendency to do

Genetically, *green squares* have a thick epidermis and thin, sparsely vascularized skin. The lack of oxygen in their skin causes them to have problems such as premature expression wrinkles, milia (tiny whiteheads), hyperpigmentation spots, cellulite, stretch marks, or scar tissue that does not heal well.

Generally speaking, *green squares* tend to neglect their health—they tend to have back problems, constipation, or arteriosclerosis—and their skin. They are also capable of being excessive in the other direction, of fanatically worrying about their health. One way or another, they always exaggerate.

Green squares will argue that they do not have time, or are not convinced. They need to see the results of clinical trials before doing something. For instance, they want to see photos of the results obtained before trying high-technology methods, such as IPL, LED, or Velasmooth laser, which others may recommend. They often want proof. They would even like to see trials on themselves before deciding.

Salespersons or counselors who cannot answer the *green squares'* questions do not sway them. Their tendency is to buy only things or services that are backed up by scientific research, logical demonstration or that can show proven results. Only a competent authority, someone who really knows what they are talking about, can convince a *green square* to do something. In general, *green squares* trust doctors and willingly follow their advice, as long as it is based on well-established facts or if it involves a program that has been specially designed for them.

What they should not do

When skin problems appear, you have got to convince *green squares* that a treatment is appropriate by presenting one or another study. But that is not all. You also have to make sure that they do not use something that is inappropriate for *green squares*, such as an oxygen-based topical application product for stimulating cutaneous free radicals.

Green squares with acne should not use what 95% of consumers use for this condition: creams whose base components are essential oils that were extracted by solvents or that contain toxic components. The solvents or toxic agents in such materials irritate and obstruct the surface of the skin with cellular debris and can cause hyperpigmentation. These substances foster the development of bacteria (such as Proprionibacterium acnes, known as PB, and Helicobacter pylori) that in turn accelerate the formation of blackheads. Instead, use essential oils extracted by distillation or maceration, which are non-toxic and non-comedogenic.

As well, *green squares* should avoid synthetic perfumes, which also stimulate the formation of blackheads and the thickening of the epidermis.

Generally speaking, of course, they should avoid any increase in stress, which provokes premature wrinkles and skin disorders, and should reduce consumption of sugar in all its forms.

What they should do

Every specific skin problem has a specific solution. But before getting specialized products to cure this or that problem, a *green square* should take the time to really understand what is specific about his or her body type and nature as a *green square*.

Let's go back to the main genetic predisposition of *green squares*: poor oxygenation of the skin at the level of the dermis. And remember the psychological trait that characterizes *green squares*: they are always jumping into all sorts of projects that causes them to live in a state of permanent stress.

These two things are related: the amount of stress a *green square* experiences directly affects the oxygenation of various levels of his or her skin.

If you want to proceed logically (which *green squares* love doing), you first have to do something about the link between stress and under-oxygenation that underlies all the *green square's* problems. The anti-aging cure for *green squares* begins with actions to reduce the stress from which all their problems originate. Stabilize the impacts of the stress that plays such a major role in their health, and you get more oxygen into their tissues—and into their lives in general.

If you can succeed in persuading *green squares* that their sympathetic nervous systems, on which too many demands are placed, are playing nasty tricks on them, then you are making important strides forward. You are helping them begin preventive work on themselves. You are helping them take action before problems appear.

If you can persuade *green squares* that:

- excessive demands are put on their sympathetic nervous systems, which therefore need to be rebalanced;
- their exercise, nutrition, skincare and interpersonal relations can serve as a major supply of oxygen, then they can switch from being their own worst enemies to being their best allies, and you will have really helped them.

They are always jumping into all sorts of projects that causes them to live in a state of permanent stress.

The amount of stress a *green square* experiences directly affects the oxygenation of various levels of his or her skin.

Autonomic nervous system (ANS)

There are several natural approaches that complement medical approaches and help regulate the activity of the sympathetic nervous system (SNS). Normally, the body rebalances the system by itself. The principal task of the autonomic nervous system (ANS) is to assure the general equilibrium known as homeostasis. The ANS constantly monitors levels of things such as oxygen, sugar, pH and adrenalin. Think of the SNS as an accelerator and the ANS as a brake.

Every time a level drops a little below what it should be for the current situation, the accelerator goes on. Every time a level goes up a little too high, the brakes are applied.

The nervous system is like an operator in a control room watching several hundred dials at the same time. Sometimes the operator reacts too slowly to restore equilibrium; he lets the reading on a dial climb a little too high before intervening. Sometime his reaction is excessive, provoking a cascade of chain reactions, for everything within the body is interconnected.

Two main possibilities threaten to disturb general homeostasis:
- the ANS does a poor monitoring job;
- the exterior situation provokes imbalances that are too important, and the ANS cannot reestablish balance.

Regulating the ANS

There are several good ways for *green squares* to regulate the action of their autonomic nervous system (ANS) to calm the activity of their sympathetic nervous system. One of these is to deepen and regulate the breathing.

- Holding your breath in a relaxed manner is a good way to bring more oxygen to the tissues. Doing so during five minutes, three times a day, is sufficient. But the best, really, is to do two minutes of relaxed breath holding when you experience some stressful situation. This can be done very discretely: during a meeting at which people are getting agitated, during legal proceedings, or in any situation that makes your adrenalin level rise.

- Another exercise consists of breathing in for five seconds through lips that are lightly pressed against each other. Let just a thin stream of air in, as if you are breathing through a straw. Because your lips are slightly closed, breathing takes a little effort. This forces the diaphragm and the other breathing muscles (the smaller pectoral, scalene and intercostal muscles) to contract more so as to draw air in. Being pressed together, the lips prevent the air being breathed out. This means you have to use your abdominal muscles to get rid of the air.

❖ The supplementary effort needed to breathe air in and out helps you become aware of your breathing mechanism.

❖ Another exercise consists of breathing in and out with your mouth wide open, as if you were yawning. Obviously you should do this exercise when you are alone, and not in public.

❖ When you yawn, the throat (or, to be more precise, the larynx) drops and enlarges to its maximum size. It is as if your throat doubles in volume. As opposed to the previous exercise, air enters the body noiselessly. The fact that the larynx drops and enlarges often triggers a yawning reflex, which will help you relax and breathe in more deeply. You should begin this exercise, therefore, by pretending to yawn, and you will find that it often ends with a genuine yawn. All this helps you digest your food.

❖ By doing five respiration cycles, with the jaw and throat well open as described above, you take in a maximum of oxygen in very little time.

Oxygenation of the skin

Our goal, in this exercise, is to oxygenate the skin by improving the superficial blood flow.

❖ To get rid of the dead skin that *green squares* tend to accumulate, they should regularly, once or twice a week, use an appropriate exfoliant. Some gentle enzymes can be used daily. Some exfoliating products are microencapsulated with alpha hydroxy, tartaric (fruit), glycolic (cane sugar), or lactic (goat's milk) acids. The acid concentration should not be greater than 10% and the pH lower than 3.5. Better still, use gentle enzymes.

❖ Here is a very simple and effective way to oxygenate the skin. Take a massage glove or a brush with natural bristles (horse or boar) and rub yourself all over, directly, without any lubricant, just once, not twice. (Repeated brushing could cause local imbalances on your body.) It is no use brushing hard. The motion of the glove or brush can be vigorous and effective without being painful. The intention is to oxygenate your skin and make you feel good. Rub yourself with the glove or brush in a counterclockwise direction, going from the extremities towards the head, starting at the bottom of your body and moving towards the top.

- There are numerous topically applied products that are designed to stimulate blood circulation. You can use them after using the massage glove or brush. The products of interest are those that contain caffeine, guarana, ginko biloba, ginseng, essence of sage or wild mint, menthol, borage seed oil, essence of cypress, eucalyptus, or bitter orange.[8] Products with a base of retinyl palmitate (vitamin A) are also recommended.

- You can also stimulate cell regeneration (mitosis) with anti-wrinkle products, stimulate the production of collagen with firming products, or unify and thin out the skin layers with lightening lotions.

If the skin is to perform its function of providing natural protection, these series of weekly treatments should be undertaken only once a year and should not last for more than a total of three consecutive months.

Green squares can have microdermabrasion treatments, once every six weeks, carefully respecting the natural rhythm of the skin. Having this kind of treatment too frequently can lead to an imbalance. Oxygenating the skin is a worthy goal, but do not overdo the cure. For *green squares*, treatments with grapefruit enzymes are too harsh and phenol peelings are often too strong. It is best to seek the advice of a skin specialist.

Sometimes, in extreme cases, only radical solutions work. Only doctors can provide these radical solutions, which require prudence. For instance, skin that appears hopelessly and prematurely aged due to too much sun exposure can be treated by a CO_2 laser, which will burn off all the epidermis. However, the skin will look burned and will take several weeks to return to its normal state. The results are surprisingly good, but the treatment is hard to endure.

---

8. Pregnant women should strictly avoid essence of bitter orange.

Exercise 6.
Muscles and angles

As in the previous exercise, we are looking for several people of the same type: *green squares*. Go some place where you will be able to observe dozens of people.

❖ Following the usual sequence, identify people classed in the family of angulars.
❖ Among these angulars identify those whose complexion is more green, with well-sculpted muscles and ideal proportions: that is, identify those who, without a shadow of doubt, are classed as *green squares*.
❖ Point by point, review the characteristics of this type for each of the subjects that you have clearly identified.
  • Color palette
  • Forms and proportions of the face
  • Forms and proportions of the body
  • Distinctive signs
❖ Note the aspects that match the type, as well as those that suggest another type. Pay particular attention to the ideal proportions of the body and to how the muscles are defined.

A lot of pure types exist in books. Reality is often more complex. The goal of this exercise is to draw your attention to a particular type and to review the type characteristics one by one, without blurring any of the differences that make each person unique.

Duration: 30 minutes

Preventive approaches

Let's come back to the question of preventive approaches. Taking vitamin supplements is one way to look after your skin. The goal of taking specific supplements is to prevent hyperpigmentation and to facilitate the absorption by the intestinal wall of B vitamins and of minerals. To this regime, you can add 1,000 to 2,000 mg of vitamin C per day, or a 500 mg tablet every three hours to reach that amount, and 1,200 mg of Omega-3, -6 and -9 per day.

Finally, a body wrap with essential oils or algae such as fucus or bladderwrack is recommended, at least once a month, both to tone the surface of the skin and to regulate the nervous system.

Green squares should remember that skin problems are linked to stress and to nervous hyperactivity. Whenever possible, relaxing activities should be combined with treatments that oxygenate the skin either from within, by ingestion, or from outside, by light therapy.

With their logical, results-oriented bent, *green squares* appreciate this complete approach of both treating the superficial symptoms visible on the skin and the deep-seated cause, the imbalance of the nervous system. They quickly become convinced that the way to get the best results is to combine various treatments.

Finally, coffee and sugar stimulate adrenalin, as you know, so reduce consumption of both.

Coffee and sugar stimulate adrenalin, as you know, so reduce consumption of both.

Interpersonal communications

Within the couple

We are going to discuss some consequences of being a pure *green square*. When *green squares* are in imbalance, some of their psychological traits become so pronounced that life as part of a couple becomes difficult.

Your partner probably thinks that it is your fault that the two of you do not communicate well and that you do not pay enough attention to him or to her. You have to admit that you do not like change, and that you are quite happy with the way things are.

There are three good reasons for this:

- Since you are autonomous and independent, you do not really need the relationship so you take it for granted and do not really pay much attention to it. The only time you do anything about it is when, from your point of view, it is not working. Caring for the other person is not your priority.
- Generally, you take everything for granted. What is the point of fussing about something that is not a problem right now? At some time in the past, you succeeded in winning your

You are autonomous and independent, you take everything for granted, and you put yourself in the center of everything partner's affection. That is done. You are faithful and you expect fidelity in return. Unlike *red ovals*, you are not looking for anything beyond that. If you do not pay attention to your partner, it is because you are got other things to think about, such as the numerous projects in which you are usually engaged. You think that your partnership is a success and that your life is under control. The idea of divorce horrifies you. And, besides, you would not have enough time...

❖ It is natural for you to put yourself in the center of everything. You are just not in the habit of seeing the world from any perspective but that of the center. You make decisions that affect the two of you without even asking your partner's advice, as if his or her assent was guaranteed in advance. Do not be surprised if, sooner or later, your partner accuses you of wanting to control everything.

It is always your excessive strength or excessive weakness that gets you into delicate situations. So what should you do? There is only one solution. You have to temper your excesses and reach a state of balance. Yes, but how?

Making better use of your qualities

Since you are so good at organizing, why not pencil into your agenda some time for your partner and your family? Plan on one evening a week. Go out together to a restaurant or to meet friends. Take time to live. Amuse yourself. Try activities, such as going out dancing or to the theatre, that may not appeal to you initially but that do please your partner. I guarantee you will feel better after such an evening than you have ever felt before.

Take the time to live

You like innovation. Encourage it in your partner. Welcome new ideas. With your partner as your guide, get out of your familiar rut. Let your partner take the space he or she needs and help you discover worlds that you find very exotic, such as Thai food, traditional Japanese theatre, or Australian aboriginal music. You will be happy, later, when you can tell your circle of friends or your colleagues at work about these discoveries. What is more, you will be seen as an interesting person.

Learn to control your impulses. Think seven times about what you are about to say before you say anything. Take a good long breath before responding.

It is always your excessive strength or excessive weakness that gets you into delicate situations.

Be there for your partner

Learn to do one thing at a time with your partner. The relationship between two people in a couple is made up of daily interactions. Leave your multiple projects back at the office when it is time to be part of a couple. Take the time to look into your partner's eyes for a minute, twice a day. These two minutes of intense togetherness will do a lot of good for your partnership and, as you will see, will allow you to breathe slowly and regularly.

Observe your partner

Observe how your partner takes care of you. Look at what he or she does to give you pleasure or to please you, and do the same. Your partner is surely not a pure *green square* like you. Two *green squares* together in a couple generally fight. Unless they really know and understand their true natures, they will not be together very long. Or they will live together for a long time, frozen in their routine, loyal to each other, but always unhappy and always in conflict.

Your partner probably knows more about looking after a relationship than you do. Do as your partner does. Then take the initiative, using one of the strategies that you have observed your partner use. You have seen your partner be relaxed and charming. Imitate him or her. If your partner is a *red oval*, you can be sure that your marriage will be a happy one. Aside from their tendency towards impulse buying, if you let your partner make decisions for the two of you, you will quickly see benefits.

At work

You like occupations that stimulate your competitive spirit. You need challenges. You like initiating and carrying out projects that bring out the best in you. As an entrepreneur, director, lawyer, artist's manager, political organizer, or film director, for example, you like being the one in charge, whether it is of a team, a company, or a factory.

You like making use of your acquaintances and colleagues. "Scratch my back, I'll scratch yours," you say. Nothing is free. Everything you do must be useful and must fit into your schedule of tasks. To forge ahead, you do not need the approval of others. All you need is your own approval. But you are demanding and hard to please, and you set very high standards for yourself.

You aim for, or occupy, a managerial position, or you act as if you are the boss. You are an ambitious, authoritarian, perfectionist, focused on yourself and your work. You easily become excessive.

When you are in imbalance, when your character traits become too pronounced, you become excessive in the following ways:

- You explain too much. You get into details that show your complete mastery of a file but that do not really help others.

- You demand too much. You are hard on yourself, and you are hard on others. Why not take a break? Allow yourself, and your employees, a break. It is not really that much time. Your comments are always about the work that remains to be done, and never about what has been accomplished. Congratulating your staff for work well done is not your style. You have difficulty saying, "Bravo!"

- Since you do not tire as quickly as others do, you do not take rest breaks. Ah! If only there was a pill to replace meals, you could gain some time and concentrate on what is really important.

- You breeze into places. You let off steam too often. It is as if the world is turning around you. Because you are too brusque and often too direct, you can hurt people.

- You are stubborn. You are so convinced you are right that it takes a really good argument to change your mind. Moreover, when you are in imbalance you are not always fair. For example, if someone proves that you are wrong or poorly informed about something, you contradict him or her and launch into a counteroffensive. This is how you behave in general: with exaggeration. Nonetheless, though you do not show it, you do notice what was said to you.

- If a friend or assistant reminds you that it is such and such a person's birthday, you pretend you remembered and did not need to be reminded. When you make a mistake, you always have a good excuse. It is hard for you to acknowledge in front of others that you were wrong and to say that you are sorry.

- You think of yourself as someone on the rise, superior to others and with an answer to everything. This attitude is not going to win you a good reputation on work teams.

- A pure *green square* is one of the biggest manipulators around. Whether you are the boss or an employee, you are constantly pushing others to do things for you. Let's take a typical example. You are a salesperson and you have been sent to a commercial show to work at a display booth. You do not think that enough money has been allocated for meals, even though you yourself do not really like stopping work to eat. You complain to a *red oval* colleague and suggest that the colleague bring up this issue at the next departmental meeting. The colleague grasps the problem, fights the battle for you, impulsively gets carried away and goes so far as to contradict the big boss in front of everybody. Result? Your colleague is reprimanded, while you stay mute in your corner. You do not even raise your voice to defend your colleague. You prefer to keep your future secure and to enjoy the good opinion of your boss.
- From what others ask you to do, you select those tasks that suit you, and you ignore the rest. You may have the intention of doing them, but you do not accomplish them. And when your colleagues finally notice, it is too late.
- You like people to be punctual. You are visibly grumpy if someone is late for an appointment or a meeting, but you are sometimes late yourself.
- Either you put pressure on the people you deal with to sign some contract rapidly, or else you read a contract many times, looking for some little glitch when there are not any. And yet, you yourself are responsible for some very messy contracts indeed.

What they should do

What should a *green square* do to improve relations at work?

If you are in management, your colleagues are going to be hesitant about giving you advice. You are generally faster than others at finding solutions. Moreover, you are convinced that you owe your position and your power to this speed.

If you are in middle management and you want to get ahead, the first thing you need to do is to learn to speak slower and to exaggerate less.

The second thing you need to learn is to relax. There is no doubt that relaxing is the best way to become more effective. As any athletic coach will tell you, the best athletes are not the most

You are generally faster than others at finding solutions.

muscular but those who know how to put themselves into a highly fluid state, to eliminate all mental resistance and useless physical tension, and to exert optimal effort rather than minimal effort.

Here, then, is what you are going to do:

- ❖ Cultivate your qualities. Indulge yourself by tackling the most complex problems and biggest challenges, or by having others assign them to you. Tackling challenges is what you naturally enjoy doing. Why not use your abundant energy and courage in situations in which others are rather timid? Give yourself the pleasure of making plans, of establishing and respecting priorities. And you will only be happier if you learn to pay compliments to all the men and women who achieve great things with you.

- ❖ Respect your equilibrium. If you ask too much of your nervous system, you are going to age faster. Heed this advice: do not take on too many projects at the same time. See each project through to completion. There will always be more interesting projects to do. It may be fun to grab the ball and run with it, to convert everything that happens around you into an opportunity, but it is not very realistic. In taking on too many responsibilities, not only do you subject yourself to unnecessary stress but also, and most importantly, you set yourself up for premature aging.

- ❖ Do not anticipate everything in detail. In succumbing to the paranoia of perfectionism, you prevent yourself from completing the big projects close to your heart. Stop organizing what everyone should be doing at every moment. Stop trying to get everyone around you to fit into your system and then, when you feel like it, changing the system.

- ❖ Learn to manage your own priorities.

- ❖ Breathe, breathe, and breathe again. Your best ally is oxygen, which is indispensable and free. If you breathe calmly, you will finally give your colleagues a chance to breathe too. Neither you nor your colleagues are robots. You know, deep down, that you are capable of listening. You know that confrontation is not the only way to get things done quickly. You know that, most often, the solution to a problem becomes obvious when you welcome the opinions of your colleagues and do not feel attacked because their opinions differ from yours. You know all this, but you tend to go to extremes and do not really pay attention to what you know.

- Make space inside yourself. Fill up your thoracic cage. Give your heart some room. You will see that a committed heart is as reliable and robust as a flawless argument. You will see that if you support the interests of others, they will support your leadership rather than challenge it. You will see that a team that pulls together is much more effective than a team that just knows how to obey. It won't take you long to realize that a team that is well-nourished, that knows to take breaks and to exchange points of view about everything concerning work, has a stronger sense of belonging, a clearer identity and a genuine pride in their achievements.
- Practice listening when communicating with others. When a problem arises, there are four questions you should ask:
  - What exactly is at issue?
  - What are you feeling?
  - What is the most difficult thing for you in this situation?
  - What resources do you have to solve this and what resources do you lack?
- The next time that a problem occurs, try to ask these four questions. You will be surprised to realize that, most of the time, people want to talk about what happened and what they thought about it. You will see that, in expressing what they felt in their hearts, they enable you to see things through their eyes. You will see that in stressing what was hardest for them, they will help you to identify the most serious problems and to draw up a list of priorities. You will realize that there are perspectives other than yours and that it is good to review all viewpoints before making a decision. You will realize that others often have a very precise idea of what they need. Most of the times it is the people on the spot who know best what to do. Most of the time solutions imposed from above are not appropriate to the actual situation because these four basic questions have not been asked. There is a time for listening and a time for action. And the rest of the time, for you, is time for breathing.

Within the family

In general, you like children, both your own and other people's. Yet you show some contradictory attitudes within your own family.

- To your own children, you are a tough and demanding parent yet, at the same time, you love them a lot and do your best for them. You make their beds for them and fasten their shoelaces, because things get done quicker and better when you do them yourself. Your kids would really like to learn what you know, because you know so much, and they admire you for your knowledge. What if, instead of always being in a rush to get everything done, you took the time to show them how to knot a shoelace properly or how to change their beds? Then you would not have to do so many things for them, and you would have more free time to spend with them. Not to mention that you would be doing them a service by letting them manage on their own.

- When it comes to school or sports, you set very high standards. You often tell them that you are not happy with their results. When they are not around to hear you, however, you boast about what they can do and make all sorts of excuses for them if they have not succeeded in some discipline. Let me give you a tip. Tell them, directly, what you say about them to your friends. It is always nice to get compliments, and they will be even sweeter coming from you.

- You play with your kids while also cooking or answering the phone. You do everything in an intense way, but you are rather impatient and very scattered. You should know that what your kids want, above all, is to be with you when you are with them! Since you are so attached to your agenda, plan some time when you will be completely available for your kids. Tell them that they can count on you at these times, which are especially reserved for sharing their company. In other words, since you like being organized, then organize some time to relax with your kids. Turn off your cell phone and plan outings, because when you are out with your kids, and no one can reach you, they will have you all to themselves. And when you are with them, do not hesitate to close your eyes and let them guide you. After all, they are the experts in the world of make-believe.

Your children are better at relaxing than you are. Why make them apprehensive by raising your voice? Why stress them out, when really you should be modeling yourself on them? They can get you to relax. They just want the best for you. They know very

You should know that what your kids want, above all, is to be with you when you are with them!

well that behind your authoritarian facade there is a big heart. They also know that hiding behind your Superman or Wonder Woman is someone who needs some rest.

Stop thinking that everything can be perfect, including family life. Stop thinking that your kids should always succeed in everything. When they are at home, they do not want to feel that there is an exam to pass. Above all, they are delighted when you do notice their A's and not just their C's.

They want to feel safe and relaxed. They want to be with adults who protect them, encourage their games and creativity, and place clear limits on their childlike behavior, but who also know how to relax and laugh with them. Above all, they need parents who appreciate them and forgive them their foolishness.

If you act like a perfect mother or father, always right and never tired, you risk making them feel incompetent relative to you. Though they try their best to please, they rarely succeed. If they feel they are not good enough, they will form a negative image of themselves, and they might even go so far as to ask themselves if life is worth living.

Family life is not about performance but about love, safety and confidence. Show them that you love them and want them to feel appreciated. Be Wonder Woman or Superman if you want to, but do so in order to make them feel confidant, not to prove to yourself that you have reached perfection.

Case study: *green square*

Enough is enough!

1st consultation

Louise was a 40-year-old physical education teacher. We met during a consultation day that I gave at a medical center in New York.

She had quite visible brown hyperpigmentation spots on her cheeks. She felt that she was in good physical shape. She was a vegetarian and paid close attention to what she ate. She exercised regularly. "So what am I doing wrong?" she asked me. She seemed skeptical. She was looking for a convincing explanation and not for a list of products to buy. I replied that I was quite happy to inform her.

She said that she had already met with an esthetician and with a dermatologist.

She had been advised to use whitening creams. In fact, these creams helped for a while, but as soon as she increased her exposure to sunlight, the brown marks reappeared on her face.

In general, her skin appeared grayish and lifeless, as is often the case for those under stress.

We began by assessing her health.

She complained of two physical problems:

- ❖ A problem of elimination (constipation).
- ❖ A problem of cellulite. Although she had an ideal figure, cellulite was clearly visible on her thighs. This cellulite was compact, fibrous, and looked like an orange skin or like cottage cheese.

She told me that she always had several projects on the go at the same time and liked living like this. She felt under pressure, she said, but in control. I told her that she had the kind of tired-looking skin that is typical of people who do too much.

- ❖ I mentioned yoga and she told me right away that she does not have time for another activity. She added that, in her opinion, yoga is a pure waste of time.
- ❖ I also talked to her about therapeutic baths with calming essential oils, massage and relaxation. I concluded by telling her that what she needed most of all was to allow herself time to take it easy and do nothing.

From that moment on, I began to have her full attention.

- ❖ I then gave her my opinion as to why her skin had a grayish color. In linking her skin, constipation and stress, I told her that she probably had a problem of poor absorption of vitamin B12. She really lacked minerals such as copper and zinc, which help this absorption. I told her about the company Activa Derme and about one of its products, called ActivaCalm (or, in Canada, ActivaBalance). Her reaction was immediate: "I don't want to buy anything." I replied that she did not need to, but she should let me continue my explanation.
- ❖ I told her that her brown hyperpigmentation spots were one of the symptoms to which she is genetically predisposed. Her body could have chosen another symptom to show its fatigue, but chose this one.

I returned to the question of the gray tint of her skin, so that she could become aware of another of the aging symptoms that affected her. I spoke to her about an exfoliant containing natural enzymes and about a cream to counteract the effects of brown marks.

She changed the subject. "Why do I have cellulite?" she asked. I explained to her that it was caused by her nervous system and by her poor assimilation of fats and her poor oxygenation.

As to her colon, I advised massages with gliding, kneading and vibratory strokes.

For her cellulite, I recommended that she try two types of massage that can break down the connective tissue, beneath her epidermis, that had become fibrous.[9] She might try:

- Manual massage;
- The kneading and infrared approach, which combines lifting and heating the cutaneous tissues by infrared light and radio frequency.

I added this recommendation:

- Using a horsehair massage glove, massage the entire body every day in a counterclockwise direction beginning at the bottom of the body. Massage in a clockwise direction in the stomach region. At home, this treatment can be followed by an anti-cellulite bath (stimulation of the blood circulation) followed by application of a cellulite cream to moisturize your skin after the bath.

I added that there was no need for her to do any weight lifting, but that she should do cardiovascular exercise and that she should drink lots of water: an 8 ounce (225 ml) glass for every 10 pounds (4.5 kg) of weight.

I ended with a couple of words about the four body types and the need to adapt her eating, exercise and skincare to her particular body type.

Louise had said she would not buy anything, and she left the consultation without buying anything. She did, however, take notes and told me that she was interested in what I had to say about her body type. She gave me her e-mail address and I sent her some documentation on body types.

---

9. These fibers have little elasticity and are perpendicular to the dermis. They deform the surface of the skin, creating the so called mottled "orange-skin effect."

2nd consultation

Eight days later, Louise returned to the clinic. This time she was prepared to try some of the products and services I had recommended. Her skepticism had begun to give way to confidence.

I noticed that there was a good deal of dead skin on her face. I asked if I could test a gentle exfoliant cream on the back of her hand.

"You won't find a single dead cell on my body," she told me bluntly. "I brush my skin every day."

The test, nonetheless, was quite convincing. I used some Soft Face Bio-Peeling, a Méthode Physiodermie product. After five minutes, when I exfoliated her skin lightly to remove the product, it came off in rolls that were unusually black. I could see that she could not believe her eyes. But, as *green squares* often do, she yielded gracefully before such irrefutable proof and decided to accept treatment with a gentle exfoliant and with an anti-brown mark face cream.

3rd consultation

Three weeks later, the brown spots were much less visible. Photographs taken at the end of the third consultation, when compared with those taken during the first consultation, showed that her skin was already better hydrated, appeared less gray and that the spots were reabsorbed. Her complexion was brighter and there were no more dead skin cells. Louise told me that this time she understood. She admitted that she had a problem and told me that she was prepared to do whatever was necessary to combat the various symptoms of aging that had appeared on her. She trusted me now.

I learned that later she had received massage treatment for her cellulite, followed by 20-minute wrappings. The cellulite greatly decreased and her thighs became smoother.

Games

3. Who has these character traits?

Identify the type to which these character traits most likely belong:

1	No matter what is going on, I know where my interests lie.	
2	I can quickly become really enthusiastic about someone or something and lose interest just as quickly.	
3	I do not have much social ambition. The most important people for me are my family and my intimate friends. It is with them that I want to spend my time. I want to help and support them in what they do.	
4	I know what is trendy and I want to be up-to-date. I do not like things that are out-of-date.	
5	I like things that are exclusive and rare. If everybody is wearing it, I have absolutely no interest in it.	
6	I have a fiery personality.	
7	I am nervous and timid.	

Answers

1. green square 2. red oval 3. white circle 4. red oval 5. green square 6. red oval 7. yellow rectangle

4. True or false?

Read the following sentences and indicate whether they are TRUE or FALSE.

Red ovals		True	False
1	Like the latest fashions.		
2	Flush easily when they drink wine.		
3	Perspire a lot when they exert themselves physically.		
4	Are predisposed to develop expression wrinkles.		
5	Are not easily influenced.		

Green squares		True	False
6	Like being told what to do by others.		
7	Like undertaking several projects at the same time.		
8	Like to have fun and are always laughing.		
9	Are predisposed to develop expression wrinkles.		
10	Are predisposed to develop brown spots (hyperpigmentation).		

Yellow rectangles		True	False
11	Like safety.		
12	Like learning all the time.		
13	Tend to be chubby.		
14	Like speaking in public to a large audience because they are extroverts.		
15	Have sweaty hands and cold bodies.		
16	Are more intelligent than the average.		

White circles		True	False
17	Are genetically predisposed to be skinny.		
18	Are not inclined to do volunteer work or to be family-oriented.		
19	Are modest, but they are also stubborn and reach their goals.		
20	Are really attracted by sugar (fast or slow).		
21	Are not good at detail and order, nor are they patient or precise.		
22	Never have swollen or painful legs.		

Answers

1. True 2. True 3. True 4. False 5. False 6. False 7. True 8. False
9. True 10. True 11. True 12. True 13. False 14. False 15. True 16. True
17. False 18. False 19. True 20. True 21. False 22. False

Yellow Rectangles
Physical exercise

What *yellow rectangles* have a tendency to do

Yellow rectangles tend to begin things but never finish them.

At the first visit to the gym, for example, they will try all the machines: the treadmill, the stationary bikes and the muscle-toning devices. They do not want to be seen as ignorant novices. They will try weights that are too heavy for them. They will play with the buttons, invent new ways to use the machines and get them jammed. If they are alone, they will ask the person in charge a lot of questions.

They act this way because they are insecure. In fact, they would like a trainer to tell them what to do and, given a strict program, they would follow it. Left to their own devices, however, they have no discipline.

They have a tendency to be extremely competitive in sports. Whether playing tennis or squash, or biking on the road, what they care about is winning. If they are beaten they suffer cruelly, and they remember such defeats for years. Even if the pride of a *red oval* can be hurt, of all the sore losers, *yellow rectangles* are the worst.

What they should not do

It is best that *yellow rectangles* not begin working out at the gym by themselves. Asking a trainer for advice will cost them more, but will give them a program that is both clear and adapted to their needs.

It is better that they avoid individual sports that are violent or highly competitive in which they might get injured.

What they should do

It is generally recommended that *yellow rectangles* do exercises that will make them slow down and breathe.

Good things to start with are meditation, isolation relaxation, or yoga.

It is generally recommended that *yellow rectangles* do exercises that will make them slow down and breathe.

They have to learn to rebalance the two parts of their autonomic nervous system, the sympathetic and the parasympathetic systems (see box: The autonomic nervous system ANS). They are far too heavily controlled by their sympathetic nervous systems. This leads to a cascade of physiological symptoms such as muscular tension, constriction of the intestines and capillaries, production of adrenalin, speeding up of the heart rate and irregular acceleration and deceleration of the heart rate.

Other recommended exercises:

- Aqua gym. When surround by water, *yellow rectangles* feel reassured and relaxed.
- Stretching the shoulders. Let yourself hang from a bar and let your own weight pull your body downwards.
- Opening the thoracic cage. With the hands behind the neck and elbows spread wide, breathe in for five seconds, hold for five seconds, breathe out for five seconds, do not breathe for five seconds. At each inhalation, push the chest forward while pulling your elbows back. Relax all the muscles you use to inhale while holding your breath for five seconds. Then breathe out during five seconds. After emptying your lungs of air, hold your breath during five seconds. Then let the air come in to your lungs by itself and start another cycle. Continue for a total of five minutes.
- Cardiovascular. For 20 minutes, three times a week, do some form of exercise, such as working out on a treadmill or bicycle, or race walking, to push your heart rate up to 60% of its maximum rate.
- Muscle toning. For 20 minutes, three times a week, train with light weights. The muscles of *yellow rectangles* will never develop as much as those of *red ovals*, but *yellow rectangles'* muscles do not need a lot of mass to become very strong, resistant and firm.

Nutrition

What *yellow rectangles* have a tendency to do

Yellow rectangles need to be munching on something all day and they rarely skip a meal.

Yellow rectangles need to be munching on something all day.

Why? Because they have rapid metabolisms and no fat storage.

Yellow rectangles have a weakness for chocolate. Unfortunately, most chocolate found in North America contains far too much refined sugar and little cacao, and refined sugar is not good for *yellow rectangles*.

They also have a weakness for cheese. They are like little mice, always nibbling a chunk of cheese. It is not good for them; indulging a weakness for cheese leads straight to colon problems and irregularities.

A third natural tendency of *yellow rectangles* is to avoid red meat and to follow a vegetarian diet. This can be a good thing for them since they have no trouble at all digesting vegetables and fruit, but they do have trouble digesting animal proteins.

They should make sure, however, that they are getting enough minerals to absorb vitamins, especially B vitamins, and that they eat enough foods that are rich in iron and protein.

What they should not do

They should avoid cheeses and red meats and cut down on sugars and yeasts.

What they should do

Make sure to incorporate foods high in protein and iron in your diet since vegetarians and vegans often neglect these foods, which are essential for good health. Adequate sources of protein include white meats, fish, nuts and legumes.

Chocolate consisting of 70% or more cocoa is a good natural cerebral balancer for *yellow rectangles*. Their inclination to follow a vegetarian diet suits their needs well. All they have to do is follow this inclination.

My strongest recommendation has to do with their attitude towards food. They never really take time to chew or breathe during meals. They quickly wolf down their food as if they were afraid that someone was going to snatch their plates away, or as if they were eating the last meal of their lives.

It is accepted practice in North American restaurants for clients who cannot finish their meals to take leftovers home. Look closely the next time someone does this, and you will see that those who ask for doggie bags are most often *yellow rectangles*. They do

Guidelines for good eating

No matter what body type you are, you should not neglect the following:

❖ Put yourself into a state of mind appropriate for digestion (relaxation);

❖ Chew each mouthful at least 10 times;

❖ Separate proteins from sugars on your plate, and eat these two kinds of food separately;

❖ Choose cold-pressed olive oil over butter;

❖ Never eat fruit with other foods;

❖ Never drink while you eat.

so not because they care about necessarily getting full value for their money, but simply because they are afraid they will run out of food. It is also often because their eyes are bigger than their stomachs, so they ordered more that they really needed. Their insecurity, their fear of not getting enough, makes them take the leftovers for tomorrow.

My advice is quite simple. If you are a *yellow rectangle*, take five minutes to relax before each of your meals. Do the breathing exercise designed to synchronize your heart rate: that is, inhale for five seconds and then exhale for five seconds while visualizing some positive scene. You need to tell your body that it is starting a rest period, and to remind yourself that meals are made to be digested and assimilated.

Skincare

What *yellow rectangles* have a tendency to do

Yellow rectangles have a tendency to do about as little as possible. They do not really care about their appearance or about personal beauty. They will establish for themselves a very simple hygiene ritual based on natural products: biological foods with no chemical additives. They will verify that each of the few products they use has been well tested and experimentally validated, but not on animals. Novelties or new technologies do not attract them.

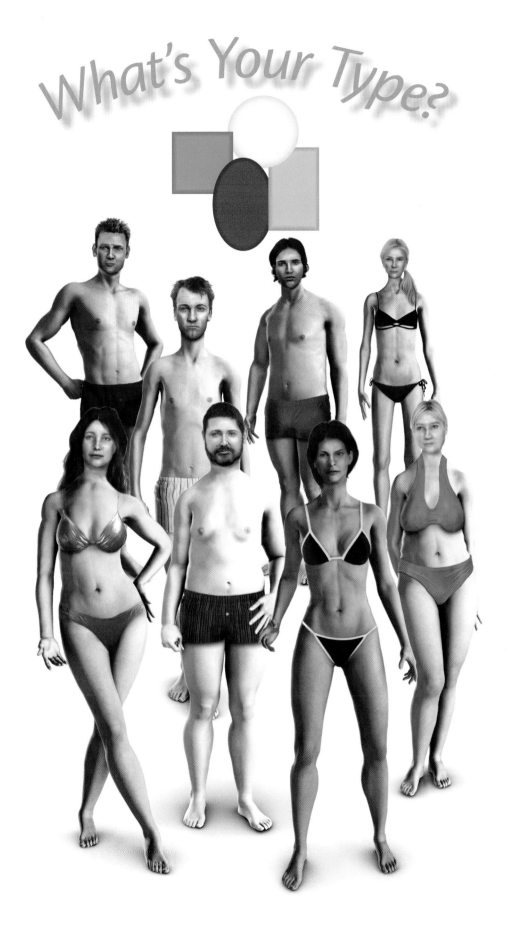

What's Your Type?

V The class of angulars

Green squares and *yellow rectangles* share certain characteristics: they belong to the class of individuals who are angular.

Shape. The angles of the body are the first things we notice in *green squares* and *yellow rectangles:* face, shoulders, waist and hips are good indicators. Their muscles are either well-defined and sculpted, or long and slender.

The color palette of their skin is yellow-green.

Their nervous systems are particularly active.

Their epidermis is thick.

The class of amples

Red ovals and *white circles* share certain characteristics: they belong to the class of individuals who are ample.

Shape. *Red ovals* and *white circles* give a general impression of roundness. They are all curves. However, even if they have a tendency to look generously shaped, do not let a mass of adipose tissue mislead you into classifying someone as ample: a *green square* can be overweight.

The color palette of their skin is red-white.

A great demand is placed on their circulatory systems.

Their epidermis is thin.

Red oval

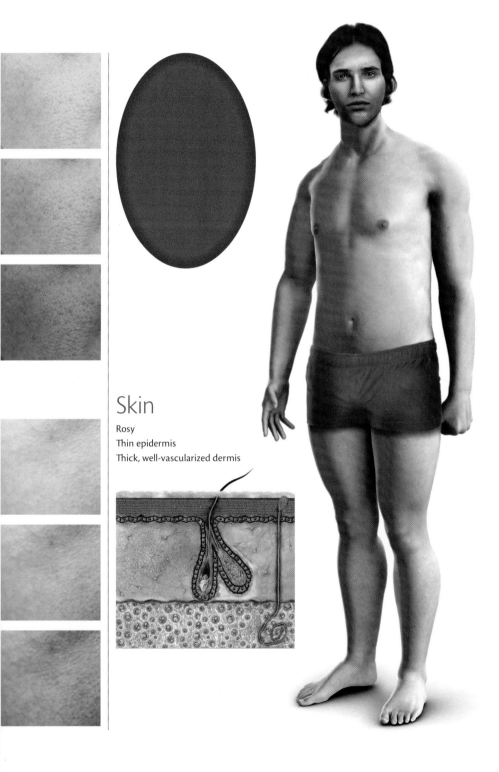

Skin

Rosy

Thin epidermis

Thick, well-vascularized dermis

Round shapes • seductive • impulsive / reactive • extroverted • energetic

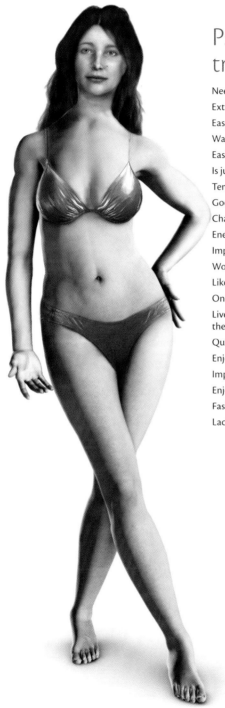

Psychological traits

Needs to be recognized

Extroverted

Easy conversationalist

Wants to please

Easily impassioned about things

Is just as quickly disenchanted

Tends towards social relationships

Good humored

Changeable

Energetic

Impulsive / reactive

Works in fits and starts

Likes to spend money

One task at a time

Lives from day to day, dreaming about the future

Quick-tempered

Enjoys being complimented

Impressionable

Enjoys good food

Fashionable

Lacks self-esteem

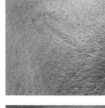
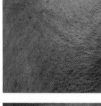

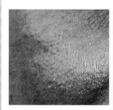
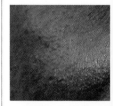
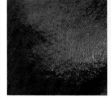

Green square

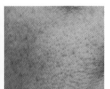

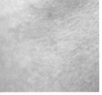

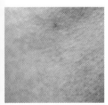

Skin

Olive

Thick epidermis

Thin, poorly vascularized dermis

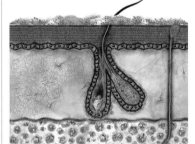

Square shapes • balanced proportions • controlling • extroverted • ambitious

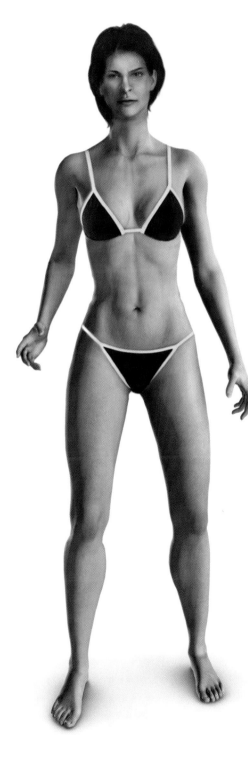

Psychological traits

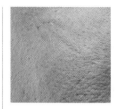

Seeks to control

Extroverted

Action-oriented

Tendency to become stressed

Plans according to objectives

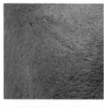

Workaholic

Likes to make money

Negotiator

Ambitious

Multitasking is normal way of operating

Lives in the future, organizes today with tomorrow in view

Autonomous and independent

Stubborn

Skeptical

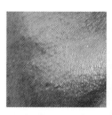

Extremist

Demanding

Egocentric

Likes to stand out from the crowd

Honest

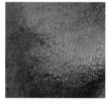

Perfectionist

Enjoys that which is exclusive

Competitive

Looks after own self-interests

Dominant

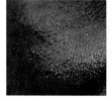

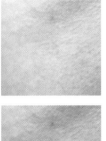

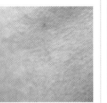

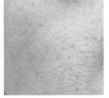

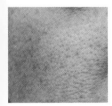

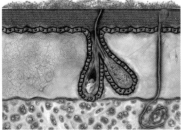

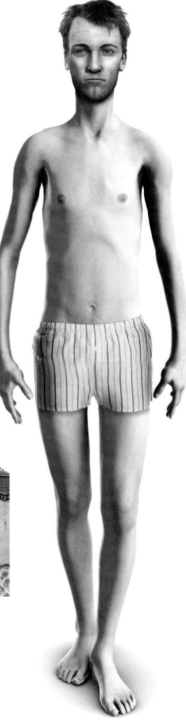

Skin

Yellow

Very thick epidermis

Very thin, poorly vascularized and
poorly oxygenated dermis

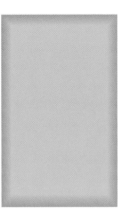

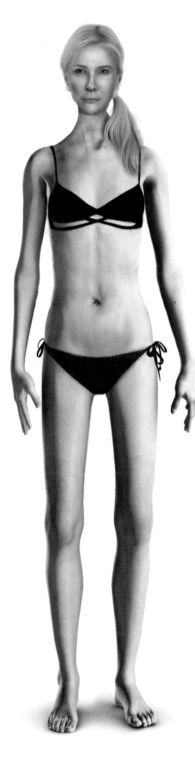

Psychological traits

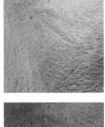

Seeks to maintain routine

Introverted

Follows others

Timid

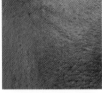

Thoughtful

Perpetually anxious and insecure

Reactive

Thrifty

Likes to be involved in several tasks at once

Lives in the past

Loyal and dependable

Responsible

Curious and enjoys learning

Opportunistic

Often illogical

Enjoys nature and animals

Plays sports

Disciplined

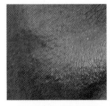

Inventive

Imaginative

Competitive, but a sore loser

Nervous

Has trouble completing projects

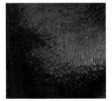

White circle

Skin

White

Thin epidermis

Thick dermis, infiltrated with water

Hypodermis contains a large number of fat cells and is filled with water

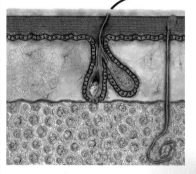

Round shapes • engorged with water • generous • introverted • tenacious

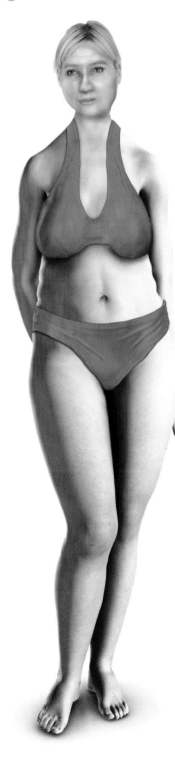

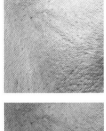

Psychological traits

Seeks to help family

Introverted

Talks a lot

Cheerful

Tends towards family or group relationships

Perfectionist who works at own pace

Tenacious

Doesn't worry about money

Works at own pace, one task at a time

Lives in the present

Has foresight

Helpful and generous

Quick to judge people

Keeps a cool head

Practical

Stubborn

Sense of detail

Precise

Loathes sports

Good, honest and dependable

Lives for others

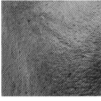

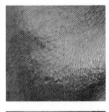

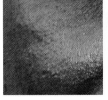

The morphological evaluation: points of reference

1 Determine the class
- General evaluation of the shape of the body and face
- Determine the palette: yellow / green or white / red

2 Determine the type
- Body shape and proportions
- Face shape and proportions
- Specific skin tone

3 Refine the evaluation
- Particularities
- Key questions
- General psychological portrait

What they should not do

Yellow rectangles are genetically predisposed to have skin with a very thin and thus poorly vascularized dermis and a very thick epidermis. They should, therefore, avoid products such as soap or creams with an alkaline pH. Their skin cannot tolerate products that have oxidized; this may happen if a tube or a jar has been open for more than a year.

What they should do

First, one has to persuade *yellow rectangles* that their skin merits more attention. The idea is not to change what they think about their appearance, but to point out that their inattention could lead to the premature development of wrinkles.

Yellow rectangles do not like being ignorant. On the contrary, they love learning. Once they understand that their type of skin needs a specific type of care, they will look after it at least as well as they look after their plants or their favorite pet—as long as the skincare product is natural and has been tested only on humans and not on animals, of course.

Three things characterize their skin:

❖ An accumulation of dead skin giving them a thick epidermis, rough-textured skin and a gray complexion. It is easy to get rid of this symptom. To help them have more supple, softer skin, they can use, twice a week, an exfoliant with scientifically well-established results. They will be surprised to see the quantity of dead cells clogging their epidermis. They will feel that they have really learned something about themselves.

❖ A poor hydrolipic balance. The cause of this problem is more deep-seated. They can clearly see the symptom of the problem—their imbalanced skin is either very dry or very oily, but is certainly less elastic (with detachment of the dermis and of the epidermis) and its surface layer is thicker—but they cannot see the deep-seated reason why their skin is the way it is. The recommended way to help restore hydrolipic balance is treatment with a detoxifying moisturizing cream.

❖ Clearly inadequate oxygenation. To deal with this problem, again, *yellow rectangles* have to be made aware of its cause.

Three things characterize their skin: an accumulation of dead skin, a poor hydrolipic balance and clearly inadequate oxygenation.

Their dermis is too thin and does not have enough room for healthy capillaries. This is why their skin often looks dull and asphyxiated. If they do not do anything, they will always have this skin tone. However, they can attain better circulation in the blood vessels that exist. As a preventive measure, it would be good idea for *yellow rectangles* to use an anti-wrinkle cream, starting when they are young, to stimulate blood circulation, a cream to increase oxygen supply and a sunscreen whenever they go outdoors. In general,

Exercises to sharpen your perception

Exercise 7.

Looking for *yellow rectangles*

Let's now move on to close observation of *yellow rectangles*. Go some place where you can observe dozens of people.

- ❖ Following the usual sequence, first identify people who are classed as angulars.
- ❖ Among these angulars, identify those whose skin is in the yellowish palette range, who have fine, long muscles and who are thin. In other words, find those who are, without any doubt, *yellow rectangles*.
- ❖ Review each of the subjects that you have clearly identified, point by point, according to the characteristics of the type.
  - Color palette
  - Forms and proportions of the face
  - Forms and proportions of the body
  - Distinctive signs

Note those aspects that agree with the classification of *yellow rectangle* and those that indicate another type. Compare the *yellow rectangles* with the *green squares* who are part of the same class. In what way do they differ in body structure? Pay particular attention to the length of the trunk and to the volume of the forehead.

Duration: 30 minutes

yellow rectangles should avoid oxygen-based products. Swedish massages are also recommended because of their effect on the blood circulation and because they help to relax. Since *yellow rectangles* eliminate little through their sweat, I highly recommend that they have a lymphatic drainage once a month. Note that the skin of *yellow rectangles* often retains wastes and toxins from metabolic activity. Such skin often forms cysts or growths around wastes that have not been eliminated. Brushing the entire body with a dry horsehair glove helps get rid of surface wastes. Using counterclockwise circular movements, begin brushing at the feet and move up towards the heart. As a precaution, use a natural brush rather than the glove on the face.

One last point. The fundamental cause of all the potential skin problems of *yellow rectangles* is their nervous hyperactivity. They have trouble believing that yoga, breathing and meditation can have an impact on their skin. Once they become aware of their basic insecurity, however, the synergy between external treatments (such as topically applied products) and internal techniques gives very good results. One should never hesitate to appeal to their mental powers, which are both their strength and their weakness. They put their entire body into imbalance through over-stimulation of their brains and of their sympathetic nervous systems; but it is with the help of these same resources that they will come to understand that they have made a mistake.

Interpersonal communications

Within the couple

The psychological traits of a *yellow rectangle* greatly facilitate life within a couple. Very loyal and reliable, a *yellow rectangle* is a partner on whom you can count. *Yellow rectangles* do not change their minds without warning. They are not like *red ovals*, who quickly tire of whatever they have. *Yellow rectangles'* sense of justice leads them to ask their partners' advice and to follow whatever rules the couple may have adopted. With *yellow rectangles*, there are no surprises. They say what they think, and they do what they say they will do. They look after their relationships on a regular basis. A bit too routinely, perhaps, yet they nevertheless enliven a group

With *yellow rectangles*, there are no surprises. They say what they think, and they do what they say they will do.

of friends. Full of curiosity, they are always discovering and promoting new artists or writers. For example, their imaginations start working overtime as soon as *yellow rectangles* start working in a field that interests them. With *yellow rectangles*, intellectual and artistic life is always sparkling.

Yellow rectangles have other traits, however, that can make life within a couple a little more delicate.

Yellow rectangles are always worried, and they like to fall back on their tried and true habits. Insulating themselves from surprises may make their minds easy, but it can make their lives monotonous. They do not get into debt but, since they keep their money in the bank, they do not profit from life. Do not count on a *yellow rectangle* to give you a plane ticket for a holiday. It is not so much that *yellow rectangles* are penny-pinching misers, but rather that they are afraid they might not have enough money in the future. *Yellow rectangles* are the kind of people who seem generous to their heirs but a little austere to their partners. In fact, *yellow rectangles* are afraid of letting themselves go, and to live with one is to live with many restrictions.

When they have to make decisions, they reflect, hesitate, cogitate and stop listening to others. Their have a taste for solitude, which can be interpreted as a lack of interest in others.

A *white circle* and a *yellow rectangle* make a good pair. The certainties of the one compensate for the uncertainties of the other. The *white circle's* desire to protect the people around him or her harmonizes well with the *yellow rectangle's* insecurity.

Here are some of the kinds of things that a *red oval* partner may say to a *yellow rectangle*. "Go on, jump into the water, you can do it!" "Forget the theory. Don't wait until everything's proven before talking about your intuitions or your discoveries." "Stop trying to control everything and make me laugh."

In an intimate and safe environment, the *red oval* may also say, "Talk to me about yourself," or, "Please read me your latest poem."

Similarly, a *red oval* may point out to a *yellow rectangle* that the air is free and good for the health, or that bending the law is not necessarily bad, but may be evidence of a spirit of freedom and fun!

As always, the point is not to change someone's nature.

Balance in a relationship comes when each partner can realize strengths and acknowledge weaknesses. *Yellow rectangles* tend to be introspective. *White circles* tend to pour out their feelings and occupy lots of space. The former are naturally skinny, while the latter easily put on weight. Both share a common love for family and children, a strong need to trust and be trusted, and a desire for family unity. Looks are not important for either of them.

At work

Yellow rectangles are full of curiosity and learn easily. Since they are often quicker than their colleagues they tend to get ahead of others and to advise everyone. Their advice is often good, but while they are helping their colleagues sort out problems they neglect their own files. It is not really negligence, though. *Yellow rectangles* have a good reason to prefer research and innovation over sticking to deadlines: they are terrified of the moment when they have to hand in their work, because whatever they do is never good enough. They are perfectionists. They think that only perfection can make them happy, and they live in fear of not achieving it. And yet, no one expects them to be perfect. They are not aware that their impossibly high standards stem from their own insecurity. No one around them imposes these standards. The people around them, in fact, admire them for their competence.

Yellow rectangles work a lot, but do not talk about their work. Their colleagues do not know just how extensive and advanced the *yellow rectangles'* work is because they do not blow their own horns. They are good at knowing things, but not at being known. They often let colleagues take credit for what they have done. They are not able to say to their boss, "This is what I did and this is how the company benefits from it." The bottom line, the difference between income and expenses, just does not interest them. Thinking up new things is what fascinates them, and they care little for final results.

Still, *yellow rectangles*, like everyone else, have to deliver the goods. It is wonderful to have a sharper intellect than others and to be able to find just the right words, but you also have to get the job done. It is one thing to have the last word in a discussion, and quite another to meet a delivery deadline.

As part of teams, *yellow rectangles* work well with people who are slower and less imaginative, but more disciplined. Put a skinny Stan Laurel together with his fat Oliver Hardy. As part of such a team the *yellow rectangle* will learn to say No and to focus on

They think that only perfection can make them happy, and they live in fear of not achieving it.

results; to accept that he or she knows enough to do the job at hand; and to get ahead using his or her own knowledge rather than striving for some unattainable perfection. Finally, *yellow rectangles* must learn never to exaggerate or to lie. The tendency to do so can make working life difficult for them.

Within in family

Families, especially children, are very important for *yellow rectangles*.

Families, especially children, are very important for *yellow rectangles*. Their parents, brothers, sisters and cousins provide *yellow rectangles* with the feeling of security they often lack. Within the family circle, they feel safe. In return, they invest in their families. They pay visits, ask for news of everyone on the phone and remember all the names. It is the *yellow rectangle* who knows the family genealogy tree and is usually the one who maintains it. It is the family that gives *yellow rectangles* their roots. They are often in the clouds, but family matters bring them down to earth.

The children of *yellow rectangles* have everything needed to be safe, especially a cellular phone; *yellow rectangles* will use these, at the appointed hour, to call their kids and make sure they are OK. To be up-to-date and well-informed as a parent, *yellow rectangles* will read all the good parenting books, from Dr. Spock to Bruno Bettelheim, including Françoise Dolto and Boris Cyrulnik. This knowledge does not ward off their anxieties. Even before a child is born, they will have selected the best school for the child—the one with the best academic reputation, with good security and one whose teachers the *yellow rectangle* has checked out through personal meetings!

Yellow rectangles will plan vacations with their families in detail, poring over all the guidebooks and maps available. They will try to learn a lot so that they can turn every visit to a cathedral or a museum into a lesson for their little angels, who will come home not just with memories of exotic sights and smells but with their brains stuffed with a lot of cultural baggage.

Yellow rectangles will take on the role of personal trainer for the family. There will be neither favoritism nor shirking. The *yellow rectangle* will insist that everyone make an effort and will get good results from everyone.

With their many talents, *yellow rectangles* will be the ones to encourage the artistic ambitions of their relatives and stage exhibits of their works. *Yellow rectangles* will encourage their kids to be free to the point of eccentricity in their art. They will teach their kids how to be really turned on by good painting or writing.

In teaching kids to appreciate art, *yellow rectangles* do themselves a world of good. Immersed in the timeless, symbolic and magic aspects of the arts, *yellow rectangles* forget their own concerns and worries. In singing, music and dance, what matters is only the present moment, and conventions become secondary. It is in the arts that the *yellow rectangles'* yearnings for the absolute are most easily realized; in this realm, they do not censor themselves nor fear that they will fail to meet deadlines.

In training the young, *yellow rectangles* themselves become younger.

The anti-aging method for *yellow rectangles* will integrate their nature, life style, nutrition, body care, and exercise and thus harness their fundamental resources to fight the ravages of time.

It is in the arts that the *yellow rectangles'* yearnings for the absolute are most easily realized; in this realm, they do not censor themselves nor fear that they will fail to meet deadlines.

Case study: *yellow rectangle*

A renowned stylist with a serious skin problem

Lynn is the owner of a Manhattan hair salon. As chief stylist, she has taken part in numerous hairstyling competitions and established an enviable reputation. She is a genuine and highly creative artist who sculpts with hair.

During a business trip to New York, I made an appointment with her to have a new hairstyle. We began to talk about one thing and another. I told her about my work developing anti-aging treatments based on the four body types. She had already heard about me through some of the talks I had given at a conference, so she was inclined to trust me.

Spontaneously, she brought up the question of her obvious skin problem. Her skin was as wrinkled as a withered apple. She was only 35 years old, but her skin looked like that of a 60-year-old woman. Lynn certainly did not have the kind of skin that you would expect for someone in her profession. She asked if I, in turn, could give her an appointment. I answered yes, of course, and two days later, we saw each other again.

Lynn is a tall and very thin *yellow rectangle* with fine and prominent bones. She seems to have more bones than skin. She is a stressed out, hyperactive smoker, with never a minute for herself. It was clear that her entire body lacked oxygen, and that she never took time to breathe.

I told her that there were far too many demands put upon her nervous system, and this was making her age faster than normal. She replied that, to keep in shape, she did a lot of exercise. She even added that she paid a great deal of attention to what she ate. She ended up telling me that she resembled her mother, that her problems were genetic, and that she could not do anything about them. "I'll die like this and that's all there is to it," she said, fatalistically.

It is always surprising to realize the extent to which people believe that everything is fixed and there is nothing they can do for themselves. Even people who have great careers and many reasons to be proud of themselves can feel powerless to improve their health.

I took Lynn's reaction as a challenge. I told her that she could not be my hairdresser with skin like that. This was just to encourage her to listen to me. I asked her to explain how she took care of her skin in the past. In fact, she used to do a lot of sunbathing with only baby oil to protect her skin and, as a teenager, would place metallic reflectors (pizza-plate style) to concentrate the tanning rays, as was commonly done in those days. When I met her, she had been going to a tanning salon three times a week, regularly, for several years. Moreover, to mask her skin problems, she put on makeup every day before going to work.

I told her that creams could not fix her problem. Her problem was linked to her predisposition to demand too much of her nervous system. It was this imbalance that had to be fixed first.

I advised her to begin with a really simple first step: to stop tanning and spend the time she would therefore save doing yoga, breathing, relaxing or simply drinking chamomile tea. And one more thing: to engage in social activities with her friends, but without her cigarettes. I assured her that just these simple changes would lead to significant improvement in her skin.

After this stage of detoxification, she should attack her skin problem and develop some new habits of living. I arranged to see her 10 days later, because I knew I would have to return to New York.

When I arrived at her salon, a regular client stopped me and asked what I had advised Lynn to do, because this client had already noticed the change in Lynn.

It is always surprising to realize the extent to which people believe that everything is fixed and there is nothing they can do for themselves.

Lynn told me right away that she had indeed seen and felt such changes. Her clients just could not stop asking her what she had done. A diet? A new haircut? Botox? A vacation?

She was really very satisfied. She seemed much more relaxed, younger and less tired. Since she found that doing yoga alone was not much fun and demanded a lot of effort, I simply advised her to take a group course.

We saw each other regularly during the following year. She scrupulously followed the anti-aging program that I recommended, including using the appropriate skincare products and taking dietary supplements, and all this successfully awakened her sleeping beauty.

Game

5. What's your color?
If you recognize yourself in the following descriptions, choose your color.

1	You are impulsive, joyous and talkative. You follow fashions and like to look good in public. Red? Green? Yellow? White?	
2	You worry when you have to make decisions regarding your financial concerns, your professional situation, or your love life. You are having trouble completing your latest project. You do not care about your image or clothing. You do care about animals and their rights and about the health of the environment. Red? Green? Yellow? White?	
3	You are good, honest and reliable. You are always planning ahead. You are the ideal person to plan the details of a trip. Family is a priority for you. Red? Green? Yellow? White?	
4	You are a dominant type. You like multitasking. You are stubborn and competitive. You are very skeptical and very demanding. You like things that are authentic and exclusive. Red? Green? Yellow? White?	

Answers

1. Red 2. Yellow 3. White 4. Green

White Circles
Physical exercise
What *white circles* have a tendency to do

When it comes to physical exercise, the main tendency of *white circles* is to do nothing. They claim that it is because they do not have enough time. And it is true that they are very busy—looking after others.

Generally, since they feel comfortable with themselves, they do not see the point of exercising. To get them to exercise you have to think up a strategy that will motivate them and keep them motivated.

In general, *white circles* are creatures of habit. They need a simple program that they can easily adapt to their daily routine. The important thing is to get them hooked. Once exercise has been integrated into their routine, *white circles* will work out quite willingly, because they like routine. For *white circles*, habit is almost second nature. The goal is to convince *white circles* that nothing has changed except for the feeling of well-being that pervades their bodies, especially their legs, which have become lighter and less painful.

The basic strategy consists of getting *white circles* to take part in some activity with another person—such as a child, a relative, a friend, a support group member, even a pet—that they already care about. For this reason, the *white circle's* home is the best place in which to exercise, and the best time is when the *white circle* is already looking after someone else. As with the *green square*, though for a different reason, the best solution is one in which the two things can be done at the same time. The best solution for *white circles* is for them to simultaneously exercise and work on a relationship with another person, which is what they care about most.

What they should not do

White circles are often overweight. Their muscles are large but lack tone. They should certainly not exercise rapidly or with heavy weights. Their hearts and their muscles are not ready for such efforts. There is no point in suggesting that they go to the gym three times a week, because most of the time they just will not go.

What they should do

White circles are always interested in going for a walk. If the *white circle* can use the opportunity to take the kids to the park, walk the dog, take his or her mother for a walk or run some errands in the neighborhood, then no other motivation is required!

The *white circle* will be happier walking for exercise if some other end justifies the walk, and if it has to be done according to a predetermined schedule.

Objective: get the lymph circulating

Walking is one of the few physical activities that *white circles* enjoy. The large lymphatic vessels lack smooth muscles capable of contracting and thus squeezing the lymphatic fluid into the channels through which it is eliminated. Since the lymphatic system has its source in the peripheries of the body and lacks a pump, lymphatic circulation depends entirely on body movement. It is muscular contractions, such as those of the calf muscles, that exert the pressure that propels lymph.

Walking or cycling can be done at a normal or at a fast pace. When accompanied by a partner, a *white circle* can readily take pleasure in rapid walking.

Power walking is the name given in the USA to a method of walking in which the entire base of the foot is used for propulsion. Instead of simply placing the feet on the ground one after the other, you land on your heels, roll through your instep and push off with the toes.

You can power walk in many ways: with a baby in a stroller, with a dog that needs exercise, with a neighbor who also wants to improve his or her physical condition. *White circles* will help themselves if, in doing so, they also help someone else.

Along the same lines, the following exercises with kids can be recommended:

- Run errands on your bike and bring a young child with you, safely installed on a bike seat.
- Go swimming with the kids at least once a week.
- Make a game of climbing up and down the stairs of the house, holding a child by the hand.
- With a child at your side, lie on your back and pedal your legs in the air, pretending to run. Anything that gets *white circles* to laugh and have fun will be good not only for them but

When accompanied by a partner, a white circle can readily take pleasure in rapid walking.

White circles will help themselves if, in doing so, they also help someone else.

for those around them, because *white circles* love to develop happy relationships.

❖ Play at being a schoolteacher and explain to the kids why it is important to make lymph circulate by moving the body. Do so after making adequate anatomical explanations.

Though children may well understand what blood is, this does not mean they understand what lymph is. Because of its semi-transparent pale color, lymph is usually not even noticed. To explain the realities of lymph to children, look at a blister that sometimes forms on your feet after a long walk as an example. Let the children touch the blister, with its mysterious colorless liquid, with their fingers. It is enough for them to feel this little bubble of liquid. They do not have to burst it to imagine how the liquid, in imbalance, invades the body and causes swellings.

Nutrition

What *white circles* have a tendency to do

White circles sometimes feel a lack of energy. Their tendency is always to react in the same way: by eating sugar for a boost of energy. Being convinced that sugar is good for them, they unthinkingly wolf down candy, chewing gum, doughnuts, ice cream, pasta, apple pies, etc. Unfortunately, this natural tendency of theirs will inevitably cause their sugar level to become unbalanced.

Since they know that they are chubby, *white circles* often start diets but, unfortunately, they often make the mistake of starting a protein-based diet. The result is that their livers and kidneys become overloaded and have difficulty in eliminating urea. Since these organs have many toxins to get rid of, it is easy to see how this kind of dieting actually has harmful health effects.

What they should not do

The first and only thing *white circles* should avoid is the one thing they crave: sugar. It does not matter whether it is quick refined sugar or slow non-refined sugar, the advice is the same: at all costs, you must avoid unbalancing your sugar level. This not only means avoiding candy and dessert, but also sugar-containing vegetables such as peas, corn, turnips, sweet potatoes, or carrots, and very

With a child at your side, lie on your back and pedal your legs in the air, pretending to run. Anything that gets *white circles* to laugh and have fun will be good not only for them but for those around them, because *white circles* love to develop happy relationships.

The first and only thing *white circles* should avoid is the one thing they crave: sugar.

sweet fruits such as bananas, dates, figs, mangos, watermelons and other melons.

As mentioned above, *white circles* should also avoid eating protein because their kidneys are often weak, and protein makes the kidneys work harder.

What they should do

Water

Though this advice may seem strange to people who are edematous, the best thing they can do is to drink plenty of water (not recommended for those with a heart condition). A *white circle* should always have a container of filtered water at home and should go around with a little personal bottle of water. The amount to drink per day is always calculated in the same way: the equivalent of one 8 oz (225 ml) glass for every 10 pounds (4.5 kg) of weight. For example, if you weigh 160 pounds (72.5 kg) you should drink 16 glasses a day.

It would be really wrong to believe that a tendency towards edema is linked to drinking too much water. The water that *white circles* drink regularly allows detoxification of their tissues. When there is an ample supply of water, toxins and pathogenic agents are pushed towards the lymph nodes, where they are destroyed by white blood cells. Water is indispensable for facilitating both the evacuation function of the lymphatic system and the filtering function of the kidneys. Water is an excellent diuretic.

To give the kidneys more help in eliminating water, you can also take sorrel, dandelion, parsley, zucchini, watercress, radish, or horseradish. Teas made with marigold flowers, artichoke, basil, silver birch, chicory and lavender are also helpful.

Lack of energy

The lack of energy that *white circles* sometimes feel is not due to a lack of sugar but to a lack of adrenalin or of internal stimulation. It is due to weakness of the sympathetic nervous system and to excessive action of the parasympathetic system (see box: Autonomic Nervous System, ANS).

White circles can get the energy boost that they mistakenly seek in sugars by slightly modifying their eating habits. By taking peppers or Brussels spouts, ginseng, or ginkgo, or by regularly drinking stimulating teas with angelica, green aniseed, mustard, basil,

The lack of energy that *white circles* sometimes feel is not due to a lack of sugar but to a lack of adrenalin or of internal stimulation.

cinnamon, fennel, ginger, sage, or thyme, *white circles* can stimulate their sympathetic systems and reinvigorate themselves.

Cocoa (and chocolate, as long as it at least 70% cocoa) is also a beneficial stimulant.

What is lymph?

Lymph forms between cells and slowly penetrates within the thousands of small open lymphatic capillaries in the periphery of the body. These capillaries join to form larger and larger vessels, with nodes from .1 to .2 inches (3 to 6 mm) in diameter, between the size of the head of a pin and of a small pea. The lymph flows into the subclavian veins to the left and right of the base of the neck. These, in turn, connect to the superior vena cava, which empties into the heart by the right auricle. The system for circulating lymph is thus connected to that for circulating blood, but it does not make use of the pressure variations caused by contractions of the heart. While blood takes just eight minutes to circulate around the body, it takes lymph six to eight hours to get from the extremities of the body into the blood system.

Draining the body

The prime role of the lymphatic system is to remove excess liquid and waist from all the tissues of the body. It is a drainage system; it drains the excess water from tissues.

Eliminating bacteria and infectious agents

Its secondary role is also an important one. It purifies the organic wastes that cells have thrown away and destroys microorganisms that could be harmful to health. When you have a throat infection, for example, you can feel with your fingers that the lymph nodes in your neck are swollen. They are battlegrounds for combat against pathogenic agents; they are swollen with white blood cells that absorb dead cells, microorganisms and other harmful substances. Lymph plays an important role in getting rid of bacteria and infectious agents before they can reach the blood supply.

Some wastes are transported by the lymph, but not destroyed. The blood system carries these wastes to the large internal filtering organs, the liver and the kidneys, where they are dealt with.

Skincare

What *white circles* have a tendency to do

White circles tend to simplify life. They only do the strict minimum for their skin. Their hygiene and skincare is basic: a little soap with, for women, a dash of lipstick and a touch of eye shadow and, for men, a quick shave. That is all. They are convinced that that is enough.

White circles have skin as soft as a baby's. It is hypersensitive. Generally, it reacts to everything: to sun, heat, cold and to rapid fluctuations in temperature and light. *White circles* worry about protecting those who are close to them and their families, but they never worry about protecting themselves.

The epidermis is thin and the dermis thick, because of water infiltration. In *white circles*, the hydric equilibrium is definitely imbalanced.

The water load has a direct effect on tissue. Over time, these water-logged tissues tend to sag under the pull of gravity. Moreover, flushing frequently appears. So what should be done about this?

What they should not do

Above all, do not make mistakes. It would be a mistake to propose a complicated care program, for *white circles* are discouraged easily no matter what they try. It would also be a mistake to use products that stimulate arterial circulation.

Avoid all abrasive treatments such as microdermabrasion and chemical peelings.

As with *red ovals*, products that are low in pH, such as those with an alpha hydroxy acid base, should be avoided.

Hot baths and saunas will cause the skin of *white circles* to flush and will exaggerate the imbalance in their hydrostatic pressure.

Among the massotherapy approaches, the friction, percussion, vibration and kneading motions of Swedish massage are too strong for the delicate skin of a *white circle* and should also be avoided.

What they should do

Drain the face and the entire body

Lymphatic drainage is the most suitable treatment for *white circles*.

Lymphatic drainage is the most suitable treatment for *white circles*. This treatment improves lymphatic circulation and clears excess interstitial liquid.

One can also use pressotherapy to complete the mechanical drainage. Pressotherapy works by surrounding the legs or the arms with a garment that is inflated by a pump. As the chambers of the garment gradually compress the surface of the skin, they act on the lymphatic system like an external pump and vary the pressure so as to provide better circulation.

Toning tissues

Micro-currents are a recommended way to restore tone to the tissues and cutaneous muscles. Also known as electronic liftings (Compulift, for example), these treatments can give fresh vigor to the muscles of the face used to express emotion. The ideal is to combine these with Light-Emitting Diode (LED) treatments, including yellow LED treatments.

Protect and hydrate the skin surface

In *white circles*, the dermis is saturated with excess interstitial fluid. On the other hand, the epidermis, which is in contact with the air, is often too dry.

Three products form the basis of a minimum treatment for this: a moisturizing cream, a decongesting serum and a mineralizing solution. To these three can be added a sunscreen, offering complete protection.

Detoxify the cutaneous tissues

Because they have poor lymphatic circulation, *white circles* often accumulate toxin on their skin. For this, the following are recommended:

- Baths with essential oils.
- Serums that will facilitate lymphatic neovascularization.
- Treatment for hyperhydrosis.
- Treatment for vasoconstriction of the venous circulation.

Exercise 8.

Identifying *white circles:* chin, neck, waist, solar plexus, ankles

Today let's move on to a careful, detailed observation of *white circles*. Go some place where you will be able to observe dozens of people.

❖ Following the usual sequence, first identify those people who belong in the family of amples.

❖ Among these amples, identify those whose skin is whiter and whose proportions are rounded—a round upper stomach, thickset ankles, double chin—and poorly defined. Find those people who are easily classed as *white circles*.

❖ For each of the subjects that you have clearly identified, review the characteristics of this type point by point.

- Color palette
- Forms and proportions of the face
- Forms and proportions of the body
- Distinctive signs

Note those aspects that match with the classification of *white circles* and those that suggest another type. Pay particular attention to the chin and to the definition of the waist, observe the roundness of the solar plexus, and do not forget the ankles.

Duration: 30 minutes

Interpersonal communication

Within the couple

White circles take up a lot of space within a couple. They are often the dominant party. They like to direct the relationship and interpret exchanges in their own way.

White circles take up a lot of space within a couple. They are often the dominant party. They like to direct the relationship and interpret exchanges in their own way. They love telling their other half what to do. They will spend forever explaining, as if their partner does not understand or has not had much experience of life. This is somewhat unexpected, because *white circles* generally will not have done much research to support what they say. Normally you will not find a *white circle* worrying about making a statement without having any proof to back it up. When *white circles* speak out, it is because they are convinced of what they say. And for them, that is enough!

It is not surprising then, that there is cause for friction if they happen to have a partner who is a *green square* or a *red oval*. Conversely, *yellow rectangles* cope well with a *white circle's* certainty, in that it acts as a counterbalance to their own fundamental insecurity.

You can also expect some major misunderstandings. Let me give you an example. Imagine the scene. A *white circle* has organized a family dinner. Everything is ready, the room looks welcoming, and the table is set beautifully with flowers and a small gift for each guest.

Just before everyone sits down, the phone rings. It is a sister calling who, knowing that she has an attentive ear, embarks on a long story about her latest financial difficulties. The *white circle's* charitable side takes over and, without a moment's hesitation, he or she promises to send money to help out the sister. For *white circles*, family comes first. Family takes precedence over spouses and even over the *white circles* themselves. Their partners, however, do not see things the same way at all. They believe that the couple should come first; they should make decisions together and then stick to them!

White circles never hesitate to support their families at the expense of the joint finances of the couple. This does not mean, though, that they depend on their partners to pay their bills for them. They pay their own bills. They do not like being in debt and, as a rule, avoid discussing money altogether. And they do not necessarily want to earn more, either.

At home, *white circles* think of everything. The fridge is always full, and they have well-stocked freezers. The whole household could survive eight days without anyone going hungry. This is one of the reasons that *white circles* and *yellow rectangles* get along so well. Life with a *white circle* may mean that you will never be rich, but you can be sure you will never go without. And above all, you will certainly never be short of love!

White circles like reading novels and watching romantic movies; they respond to sincere emotions. *White circles* can be naïve and sentimental in the realm of the imagination but, on the other hand, they are exceptionally practical and down to earth in daily life. If you want to make a *white circle* happy on his or her birthday, give them a toaster, a bigger and better stove, a central vacuum cleaner, a garden tool, a toolbox or a new novel! Perfume or something to please the senses simply is not even worth considering!

When you offer flowers, a *white circle* will thank you warmly, but always with, "But, you shouldn't have!" Another time, when you come armed with a plant for the garden, the look of pleasure on a *white circle's* face will show you that you have got it right. You are most likely, in that case, a *yellow rectangle* yourself with the same love of nature!

White circles will enjoy offering you a ticket to the theater and place it in an envelope with a beautiful ribbon around it. Observe how impatient they are watching you open it! This is all part of their pleasure at giving a gift!

White circles like cars that are spacious enough to hold a large number of people. With a big SUV or minivan, they are sure to be able to take everyone along in comfort and in style. There is enough room to take the kids to the pool, or over to the hockey rink, or to help out by picking up their neighbors' kids, as well as their own, after school.

There is another problem: *white circles* are hard-headed. Although they are sensitive, gentle nature-lovers, they are not very flexible! Do not try to change their vacation dates once they have been fixed. In a few carefully chosen words, they will quite firmly explain why it is impossible to accommodate any changes!

Asking *white circles* about their families is a sure way to gain their approval. Ask after their mothers or fathers. Find out if they have children, or any brothers and sisters. Ask them if they have photos of their families to show you. Remember to ask them about a recent family celebration or birthday party, or about the vacation

Life with a *white circle* may mean that you will never be rich, but you can be sure you will never go without. And above all, you will certainly never be short of love!

they have just had with their friends. Given the chance, they will simply love telling you all about their experiences. Or they will tell you about something interesting they have just found in the newspaper. Let them talk, and they will tell you what they have learned. Just listen; they will love you for that alone!

White circles are like sponges. They absorb everything that is going on around them and remember it, too. They will tell you how they feel, recount a recent conversation and talk about what is happened to them whenever they get the chance. This is how they socialize.

If the relationship starts to get rocky, if the atmosphere becomes tense, it is good to know that a *white circle* will not be in a hurry to divorce. *White circles* try their very best to find solutions. If their partner envisages a separation, they will want to talk things over in great detail. *White circles* will find excuses for partners who leave them. They stand up for everyone, even the partner who walks away. *White circles* put themselves last.

Those of you who have recognized yourselves in this last section have many of the qualities that it takes to live as a couple: you are faithful and trustworthy, your home is your castle and your family is sacred to you. You make use of these qualities every single day, and no one can doubt them. You can quite rightly be proud of your devotion.

That being said, you need to stop trying to lead your partner by the nose and being pushed around yourself. In fact, it is all part of the same character trait: the tendency you have to dominate is the other side of the coin to your tendency to put yourself last. In the same way, your habit of holding back is the same as your love of giving. In short, it could be said that you keep a lot and you give a lot or that you keep too much and give too much!

What you are consciously or unconsciously trying to do is to keep a balance between your different excesses, and you usually spend a lot of time juggling. To find balance, you will have to look on the side of minimalism. Hoard less, talk less, and give less. For once, go for the minimum rather than the maximum. First and foremost, think about yourself.

Of course, it is not in your nature to be a minimalist, but trust me; it is in your own interest to do less. Doing less will give you more time for yourself and for your family. Put this into practice, and others will see that life can go on without you. Even if you do less, you will see that there is still plenty of room for you in the

> The tendency you have to dominate is the other side of the coin to your tendency to put yourself last.

couple. You have to understand that your courage and devotion to the cause of others stem from a fear of not being loved. You will see that taking up less of the conversation time will mean you are given more room. Let me put it another way. Be sparing with your words and benefit from listening.

But how can you start? You should know that the solution to a shortage is not excess. Storing up and holding back prevents you from giving the true gift of yourself. If your partner loves you deeply, then let him or her see what is missing for you. If your partner loves your full shape, let him or her see that it is emptiness that frightens you. Tell your partner clearly that if you do so much for others and nothing for yourself, it is not because you have everything you need, but because you are afraid of being worthless. Once you have admitted all this, let your partner have a little more say at home and in the family; rather than taking away your importance, you will see the opposite. You will see your stature increase. You will soon be happy to observe the positive effects of your new attitude towards yourself.

At work

White circles find that the same qualities and limitations that mark their home lives are also seen in their relationships at work.

When they are part of a team, *white circles* have a tendency to be know-it-alls. They do not really like being told what to do. Like *green squares*, *white circles* are stubborn and want to achieve their objectives. But with one difference: *white circles* do not like having many projects on the go at once. They object to being put under pressure or being pushed at a faster pace than they would choose. Respect their rhythm and you will find they are trustworthy, faithful and good-natured. But when you push them, they will be frustrated and bad-tempered. Let *white circles* finish project A before asking them to take on project B, and all will go well. The job will be done properly down to the last detail. In the same way that nothing is missing in their refrigerators, nothing will be forgotten at work.

White circles like to take their breaks in their own way. For example, they may decide to talk to their colleagues, but it will be to only one at a time. They like seizing the opportunity to give their opinion about a project without being asked—it allows them to relax and, at the same time, lowers their blood pressure! Yet

Respect their rhythm and you will find they are trustworthy, faithful and good-natured. But when you push them, they will be frustrated and bad-tempered.

they are also capable of listening to a long, detailed explanation from a colleague expressing his or her ideas. In return, they expect their colleagues to give as much time to listening to them and hearing their ideas. But very often, their co-workers have a higher opinion of themselves and, thinking they know much better, generally want the last word. In fact, people like to confide in *white circles*, but they tend to disappear as soon as *white circles* start to behave like them!

When they train others at work, *white circles* like to show off their expertise. If you show them something, they will remember it and bring it out at a later date, but they might forget to acknowledge you. This is not because they are not grateful; it is just the way they are. Their nature is to appropriate things for themselves. *White circles* will talk about an article they are writing about a technique they use, knowing full well that it came from you or another person. *White circles* are not being dishonest, but the knowledge they draw on has to come wholly from them, even if it originated elsewhere. *White circles* retain anything that they think could be useful to them. This is how *white circles* learn—by remembering.

White circles look for jobs that will allow them to give full rein, on one hand, to their sense of detail and precision and, on the other, to their interest in human relationships. It would be ideal for a *white circle* to be an accountant and to be the volunteer head of the social committee. Or perhaps an appraiser who is also in charge of all group parties!

White circles do not find it easy to lead a team at work, because they lack determination. They have difficulty getting an overview and stepping back to see the big picture. They stick to a task, they listen, and they can recite what they have been told word for word. They remember everything about a training session that they have just attended. But generally, they do not feel they have what it takes to develop a research project or to devise a new theoretical approach to a task.

They are not the complainers in a team. *White circles* work tirelessly. You only have to ask for their help and they will give it. They will even go so far as to offer to help you out if you are running late. Yet if they experience any trouble with their own work, they will not come knocking at your door. This is not due to false pride, but because they just do not want to bother you.

Within the family

White circles are protective parents, with endless energy. They are genuinely worried about their children's health and happiness. They are always there for their children and do everything in their power to make them happy, expecting nothing in exchange. Just the joy at seeing their children's contentment is sufficient reward for a *white circle*.

On days when *green squares* do not feel well, you will not catch them pushing themselves to bathe their sons or daughters. They will rest and put the bath off until the next day. But *white circles* force themselves, somehow finding the energy it takes. They do not look for excuses; hygiene is far too important to them!

A *white circle* mother will prepare a well-balanced, nourishing picnic. She will fill the hamper with everything that could possibly be required: plates, knives and forks, of course, but she will also include a towel for hand washing, a blanket to sit on and sunscreen!

White circle fathers have infinite patience; they will show their kids how to assemble or take apart something, while in the process taking care to explain how it all works. They will take them sledding or skiing in winter. At the rink, they will be lacing up their skates and putting their gloves back on.

White circles want to pass on the values in which they believe so strongly: work, joy, respect, listening, care for details, responsibility, giving of oneself and a sense of enjoyment and sharing. All this is commendable and lovely to see.

The problem, however, lies in the fact that *white circles* have difficulty letting go. Out of earshot of the child, you might hear them saying to a friend, "I can't wait to see him grow up and leave home." But, in reality, it is not what they want at all! You might even hear them another time stating firmly, "I'm not a mother hen." "You won't catch me spoiling my kids." But that is absolutely what they are and what they do!

They will defend their children tooth and nail, as indeed they defend all their loved ones. They will tell you, "My kids have never touched drugs!" even if one of them has a drug problem. The white lie is used to protect their child's reputation even more than their own.

So *white circles*, please stop doing quite so much for your children. You need to do a lot less! Stop trying to save them from the slightest harm and to keep every possible problem at bay!

White circles have difficulty letting go.

Do I hear you saying that you do it out of love? And what if I tell you that it is also out of fear? Fear of not having enough authority? Fear of saying no? Fear, too, that they will reproach you for not loving them? And fear of seeing them leave home one day?

You prefer to deprive yourself rather than set limits to their wants and needs. You avoid putting up any resistance, you never complain. You are telling them, without saying so openly, that being a spoiled child is OK. Is this really the message that you want to give?

What about your values? What about respect? The joy of sharing? How are they going to adopt the values you think are important if they have never been required to practice them?

If they grow up thinking that your values are what allowed them to satisfy their immediate desires, there is little chance that they in turn will adopt these values when they become parents. If they watch you and see that all your efforts have gone into ensuring that nothing is required of them, then there is no way that they are going to want to imitate you!

Parents are entitled to have privacy, boundaries and their own territory. If you convey the message that the parents' job is to give their children round-the-clock attention, you will have no time or space left over for a life of your own.

The only personal space you will have is the space occupied physically by your body. Now, here are some surprising questions worth considering for a moment: Might *white circles'* roundness not be their way of taking up space? Is it a physical expression of their desire to claim the space that is theirs by right? Could it be their way of getting others to respect their space?

Case study: *white circle*

How skin problems can stem from a more generalized problem

At a conference in New Orleans, I had set aside a day for consultations at a medical clinic specializing in skincare.

A 17-year-old African-American man came in with his mother. We will call him Jermaine. The appointment was for him. Immediately after we all greeted each other, his mother took control of the conversation. She started speaking to me before I could ask any questions and, when I asked her son anything, she was the one who answered.

I observed Jermaine's skin closely and felt the skin on his forearms, his face and lower calves. I studied the general shape of this body and observed his relationship with his mother. I listened to his responses to my usual health questionnaire. Everything suggested that Jermaine was a *white circle*. He had a bad case of vulgaris acne (teenage acne), which was why he had come to see me.

Jermaine wore a ring on his right hand but his fingers were so swollen that he could no longer remove it. He complained that his legs hurt. Both legs were swollen around the ankles. His skin was gray, which may seem surprising for someone whose skin color was dark. But it was really gray, dull and lifeless. His face was round and puffy, and he had a double chin.

When I asked him what he ate, the answer came straight back; he loved anything sweet, especially candy. He said he drank a lot of milk (unskimmed) and sodas (with sugar). He ate lots of cheese and pasta. All those typical *white circle* favorites were clearly important in his diet.

We talked for a while, and I learned that the other kids were teasing him at school because of his weight and his acne. He told me that he hardly did any sports anymore because he hated the others laughing at him.

He was a pleasant, quiet boy, but rather shy. His answers were honest and he seemed to appreciate that I was listening more to him than to his mother. As she watched me working, she talked nonstop, thinking she was helping. She was answering questions and suggesting solutions, but her comments were completely off-track.

I explained to Jermaine that he had what is known as vulgaris acne. I told him that it was a localized symptom of a more generalized problem that affected his whole body.

My message was that this generalized problem needed to be addressed. Treating the acne alone would only bring temporary relief. It would never completely disappear. I told him that if he made a huge effort to eradicate the underlying problem that affected his whole body then, at the same time, he would be treating the localized symptom, which would then lessen and disappear.

Until then, his dermatologist had been prescribing a treatment purely for his acne. It was the first time that Jermaine had heard that his problem went deeper!

What was this second problem? I told him that I knew what it was: his lymphatic system was unbalanced. Then, I showed him what this meant, with the help of some examples. He quickly understood.

It was the first time that he had realized that he had a build up of fluid in his arms, legs, face and neck. He thought it was simply fat. I showed him the difference when I pressed a finger on his arm and then did the same thing on my own arm. He saw the mark left by my finger. He saw how long it took for his skin to bounce back to its original position.

The hypertoxicity of his skin was not due to any localized infection, but to bad drainage of the waste products of his body's cellular metabolism. This was the root cause of the infection we could see, his acne.

To clear up the problem, I prescribed some concrete actions for him to take, pointing out that he could not expect to get the results he wanted unless he was sure to carry it out properly. The effects would be cumulative and only by doing everything would he achieve a satisfactory result:

- Drink water. I explained to Jermaine and his mother that if you retain water, the most important thing to do is to drink one 8-ounce (225 ml) glass of purified water for every 10 pounds (4.5 kg) of body weight. He was very surprised, but not as surprised as his mother.
- Apply a decongesting serum to the skin daily. Why decongesting? He did not see the point. I explained that the serum was not for eliminating the acne, but to improve the lymph circulation. Lymph transports and eliminates the toxins in the body. When lymph circulation is inadequate, the toxins accumulate in the cutaneous tissues, causing local infection.
- Drink a diuretic herbal tea twice a day to aid the elimination of toxins in the urine. Take a natural detoxifier to aid the liver in its role as filter.
- Immediately cut sugar consumption by 50%. We talked about how he was going to do this.
- Cut consumption of cheese by 50%. I let him decide for himself how he would eat less. I approved his plan.

We then moved on to the subject of physical exercise. I did not think bodybuilding exercises with weights would be right for him. My first suggestion was that he ride his bike to school, which was a 15-minute walk from his home, or else walk there at a brisk pace.

I also suggested some isometric exercises. These consist in maintaining a stationary position for as long as it is comfortable to do so. You aim to hold the position for a little longer each day, as long as no pain is felt. An idea that I generally find works well is filling out a daily log. Showing it to friends and family, and hearing their congratulations gives a lot of encouragement.

From the wide range of possible isometric exercises, I recommended two that work on the back and leg muscles, which are generally quite strong in those who are overweight. Everyone is capable of doing these exercises for a few seconds, so no one should find them discouraging. You just need to adjust the duration of each exercise to how strong you are feeling.

What I suggested to Jermaine was to do the exercises with a stopwatch (of course) and also with a partner—his mother! She was in need of the exercises just as much as he was. And I was expecting that the exercises would put Jermaine in a position of superiority with regard to her. I felt that he needed to prove that there was something that he was better at than she was. Both welcomed my suggestion but, no doubt, for quite different reasons!

Exercise 1

For exercise 1, you have to lean against a wall, legs bent at 90 degrees, shoulder-width apart. It is a favorite exercise among cyclists, ice skaters and skiers. I told Jermaine to take time to control his breathing during the exercise. The breathing exercise is the one I have mentioned before: breathe in for 5 seconds, hold for 5 seconds, breathe out for 5 seconds. All you have to do is to stand like that without moving, keeping the back pressed against the wall. Start the stopwatch and count the seconds. The aim is to hold the position for one minute. I told Jermaine that holding for just 15 seconds the first day would establish a good record. He understood that he should stop as soon as it became uncomfortable. I told him to keep a careful record in his log book, and to increase the length of time each day. He would set his own objectives, challenging himself according to his strength. He would be his own trainer and was to show his results to others. His mother was to do the same thing.

Exercise 2

Exercise 2 should be carried out immediately after exercise 1. It prolongs and intensifies the effects of exercise 1 and at the same time allows you to relax. Lie down on the floor, raise your legs and place them against a wall. This allows the lymph to return towards the heart. Hold this position for as long as you are comfortable, gradually increasing the length of time.

The effect of both these exercises is to produce a change of pressure in the legs. The second accelerates lymph circulation, encouraging it to return to the main collector, Pecquet's cistern, and into the blood stream through the subclavian vein.

I also advised both Jermaine and his mother to complement these exercises with as many pressotherapy sessions as they could afford.

I also suggested using a bacteriostatic cleanser to treat the acne flare on his skin plus a keratolytic exfoliating cream.

Results

I saw Jermaine again two months later. He came for his next consultation, still accompanied by his mother. His skin was beautiful, smooth and healthy. He looked great.

The first thing he told me was that his schoolmates had stopped laughing at him because of his acne. Though he still had a few excess pounds to lose, he had quite clearly worked hard at the treatment, which had not only led to a real improvement in his lymphatic circulation (round shape), but had also helped his acne. In addition, his self-confidence had increased. When he proudly showed me his log book, and when I saw that he could talk to me without letting his mother interrupt, I understood that their relationship had changed. He was occupying his personal space, and she was giving him more space. He deserved my heartfelt congratulations. His mother also showed me her own log. She had obviously been caught up in the game. I congratulated her warmly too.

Exercise 9.

Use your friends: touch and feel!

It is not very often that we have a group session where we touch and feel. But, it can be very helpful. It is certainly worthwhile taking a close look at skin. No two skins are alike. They will never be the same color, texture, or thickness, and no skin gives off the same amount of heat. Today we are going to explore all the fascinating differences you can find in skin. When you do this exercise, treat it as adventure, like going on a safari in deepest Africa!

As you have probably guessed, for this exercise you will need the help of some of your friends. Three or four people should be sufficient. As you work through it, make sure that you finish evaluating one person on each point before you move on to the next. Ask your volunteers what they think and let them experiment, too. Sharing your discoveries means more fun!

❖ Look at the bare forearm. Observe the skin from elbow to wrist and all around the arm, inside and outside. While you are doing this, identify the color palette. Ample (red-white) or angular (green-yellow)? Touch the skin. You will already be able to get an idea of its thickness, elasticity and of the heat it gives off. Compare one person with another. Is their skin texture thick or rough? Does the skin feel dry, soft or rough? Why not ask your friends how they care for the skin on their arms. By now, you will have been able to form your first general impression.

❖ Now, test the capillary return on the inside of the forearm. Press the skin firmly with your fingertips. Then, quickly remove your hand and watch the reaction of the skin.
- Did the skin change color when you pressed it?
- If it did, did the original color return quickly?

❖ Now, still working on the inside of the arm, compress the skin near the elbow between your thumb and fingers.
- Is the skin particularly elastic?
- Does the dermis adhere well to the epidermis, or do you feel the layers separate from each other?
- Do you feel a build up of fluid or lymph between the dermis and epidermis? This may feel like small bubbles of water moving beneath your fingers, or you could even feel a pool of liquid under the skin.

Exercise 10.

Asking questions Columbo-style

When we do a type evaluation, the questions directed toward morpho-logical characteristics often allow us to determine the predominance of one particular body type. They are especially important when the other factors leave us undecided.

Today you are going to behave like Lieutenant Columbo. I am sure you re-member that inquisitive detective in who wore an old trench coat played by Peter Falk. With his apparently innocent questions, he always managed to deduce who was the murderer.

Do not give the game away in this exercise. Keep secret what it is you are trying to find out. You can slip your questions into the course of an ordinary conversation without awakening any suspicions. Columbo always used to mention his wife—whom we never actually saw on screen—and in talking about her, he made his clever, well-thought-out questions look anything but serious. You can try the same. Try inventing an aged aunt who suffers from a multitude of symptoms!

I recommend that you ask these three sets of questions.

- ❖ Do you feel the cold? Generally, or when you are tired, are your hands, feet, or the end of your nose cold? You will need to differentiate between those who always feel a little cold all over, and those in whom only the extremities and not the entire body are cold. The former being *yellow rectangles* and the latter *green squares*.
- ❖ Does your skin quickly turn red in the sun? Is it red and blotchy after a hot bath? Do you flush when you eat spicy food? Do you perspire easily? (Do not let this be your first question!) These questions all point towards reactions that are typical of *red ovals*.
- ❖ Do your legs hurt in the morning? Do they feel heavy or numb? People who are predominantly *white circles* will answer yes to this last set of questions. If, on the other hand, the legs hurt in the evening, it is prob-ably due to venous insufficiency, a characteristic of *red ovals*.

Be sure to ask each person the whole set of questions. Affirmative replies can con-firm the predominance of one type or indicate an important secondary type.

Anti-aging: the cure for *green squares* and *yellow rectangles*

The instructions for the treatment are set out clearly here, and you will find them simple and easy to follow. I strongly suggest that you consult a healthcare professional to help make the treatment just right for you according to your type.

Since their bodies are clearly angular, *green squares* and *yellow rectangles* can be grouped together. Neither group carries many extra pounds, their shapes are not at all rounded, and they are smaller framed.

Ground rules

- When you wake up in the morning, drink a glass of filtered water at room temperature, with a little lemon zest;
- Do five minutes of stretching, breathing exercises, or yoga;
- Do 20 minutes of cardio;
- Three times a week, do 30 minutes of the muscle-building exercises to work all the muscle groups;
- Once or twice during the day, drink an herbal tea such as ginseng, mint, or ginger.

Supplements: vitamins and minerals

Here is a list of dietary supplements. It is a good idea to take them with breakfast to ensure that they are not forgotten. The maximum dose is indicated for those suffering from an imbalance, while the minimum dose is sufficient for preventive maintenance.

- A complete multivitamin containing 5,000 international units (IU) of beta-carotene and 5,000 IU of vitamin A;

- Calcium citrate: 350 mg to 1,200 mg;
- Magnesium chelate: 350 mg to 1,200 mg;
- Silicon: 200 to 400 mcg;
- Alpha-lipoic acid: 100 mg to 300 mg;
- Omega-3, -6 and -9: 1,200 mg to 3,600 mg per day, directly in the form of 400 mg salmon oil, 400 mg flax oil and 400 mg borage seed oil, as contained in 1 to 3 capsules per day;
- Vitamin C: 500 mg to 3,000 mg per day. Remember never to take more than 500 mg at one time. Since the body cannot absorb a greater dose than this, any more will only be eliminated. However, it can be a good idea to take a dose every three hours, particularly if you are going to be out in the sun or subject to atmospheric pollution.
- Smokers should know that cigarettes create a number of free radicals and accelerate the aging process. Smoking is heavily discouraged. If you do smoke, you should take 500 mg of vitamin C every three hours.
- Selenium: 200 to 400 mcg per day;
- Vitamin B complex: 1 to 3 tablets of vitamin B complex with minerals, which should include:
  - B2: 10 mg to 30 mg;
  - Niacin: 100 mg to 300 mg;
  - B12: 12 mcg to 36 mcg;
  - Biotin (for absorption): 45 mcg to 135 mcg;
  - Pantothenic acid: 20 mg to 60 mg;
  - Folic acid: 0.4 mg to 1.2 mg;
  - Zinc: 23 mg to 29 mg;
  - Copper: 3 mg to 9 mg.

Consult a doctor to add 50 mg to 200 mg of DHEA per day to your treatment if necessary. (This is not permitted in some countries.)

Meals

Here is a typical meal plan for a day.

Breakfast

- Cereals should be wholegrain, or go for oatmeal or grains;
- An hour after, drink a glass (half a cup) of soymilk, or a glass of orange juice. Then have wild berries (blueberries, raspberries) of your choice.

Lunch

- A green salad composed of fresh bright green leaves, with an olive or onager (evening primrose) oil dressing;
- One slice of low-fat cheese (feta, goat);
- A small piece of chicken;
- A plain yoghurt;
- Dessert, one hour later, can be bright-colored fruit.

Afternoon

- Drink four to six 8 ounce (225 ml) glasses of water;
- Around 4 p.m. have a snack consisting of nuts or a banana.

Dinner

- Carrot or any colorful vegetable soup;
- Pasta with tomato sauce;
- Fresh wild salmon, or chicken;
- Have colorful vegetables, such as bell peppers, broccoli, or asparagus, as a side dish. The antioxidants and vitamins they contain are very important for *green squares* and *yellow rectangles*.

General remarks

- Never drink during a meal;
- Drink one 8 ounce (225 ml) glass of water for every 10 pounds (4.5 kg) of body weight (or about 2 glasses for every 5 kg of weight);
- Take time to relax before you eat (you may want to pray, do breathing exercises, or some yoga);
- Use first press, cold-pressed virgin olive oil rather than butter or margarine;
- Chew well before swallowing your food, to give the digestive juices in your saliva time to work;
- Opt for organic foodstuffs;
- Eat fresh vegetables within 24 to 48 hours of purchase;
- Avoid restaurant buffets (the food will often have become oxidized);
- Avoid sugar and anything containing sugar;
- Of what you eat, 80% should be bright colorful vegetables (alkalis) and 20% should be your favorite mouth-watering foods, which may include fried food, sauces, cold cuts or

grilled meat, all of which are acidic and otherwise should be avoided.

> *Green squares* and *yellow rectangles* should pay particular attention to the health of their colons.

Supplements:

- Silymarin (milk thistle): 200 mg to 600 mg;
- Dandelion root: 50 mg to 150 mg;
- Magnolia vine: 50 mg to 150 mg;
- Licorice root: 50 mg to 150 mg;
- L-cysteine: 100 mg to 300 mg
- Probiotic Lactobacillus: 1 to 2 million cells per day. Each dose is ready to be mixed with plain yoghurt.

Anti-aging: the cure for *white circles* and *red ovals*

The instructions for the treatment are set out clearly here, and you will find them simple and easy to follow. I strongly suggest that you consult a healthcare professional to help make the treatment just right for you according to your type.

Since their entire body shapes are rounded, with no straight lines or sharp angles, *white circles* and *red ovals* can be grouped together. They are not small or even medium-framed. *White circles* and *red ovals* are corpulent with large bone structures.

Ground rules

- ❖ Once or twice a day instead of coffee, drink either ginseng herbal tea, green tea, or hawthorn flower tea;
- ❖ When you get up in the morning drink a glass of filtered water with a little lemon zest.

Supplements: vitamins and minerals

Here is a list of dietary supplements. It is a good idea to take them with breakfast to ensure that they are not forgotten. The maximum dose is indicated for those suffering from an imbalance, while the minimum dose is sufficient for preventive maintenance.

- ❖ A complete multivitamin including 5,000 international units (UI) of beta-carotene;
- ❖ 5,000 IU of vitamin A;
- ❖ Calcium citrate: 800 to 1,200 mg;
- ❖ Magnesium chelate: 800 to 1,200 mg;
- ❖ Chromium picolinate for imbalanced *white circles*: 200 mcg to 400 mcg per day;
- ❖ Bioflavonoid supplements combined with vitamin C: 1,000 mg to 3,000 mg per day
- ❖ Alpha-lipoic acid: 100 mg to 300 mg per day;

- Coenzyme Q10 (an antioxidant that helps maintain cardio-vascular balance, which is very important for *white circles* and *red ovals*): 100 mg;
- Omega-3, -6 and -9: 1,200 mg to 2,400 mg per day, directly in the form of 400 mg salmon oil, 400 mg flax oil and 400 mg borage seed oil, as contained in 1 to 3 capsules per day;
- Iodine: 100 mcg;
- Garlic: 1,500 mg to 1,800 mg (alliin);
- Field berries: 80 mg twice a day for *white circles* and *red ovals* who are out of balance. Do not forget that you should be eating fresh field berries in their natural form.

Meals

Here is an example of a typical meal plan for a day.

Breakfast
- Colorful fruits (raspberries, blueberries, cranberries);
- Rye bread.

Lunch
- Fresh, wild, coldwater salmon, or chicken;
- Green vegetables;
- Avoid cheeses.

Afternoon
- Four to six 8 ounce (225 ml) glasses of water;
- Around 4 p.m. have a snack, preferably of raw fresh vegetables like celery or zucchini.

Dinner
- White meat;
- Vegetables;
- An hour later, fruit or yoghurt.

General remarks
- Increase your consumption of potassium, garlic, celery and onion;
- Never mix proteins and slow sugars during the same meal;
- Never eat fruit, including tomatoes, along with other foods;
- Wait one hour between eating them.

Colors of Benetton

Do you remember that Benetton ad that showed a group of different people all with different skin colors? Many people at the time were offended by it. But just think how many ethnic and cultural barriers have fallen since then! And these barriers are still falling. After so many years concentrating on our differences, we are now beginning to see how similar, in fact, we all are. And, in this, skin is no exception. It comes in a wide range of very different shades, but no matter how light or dark we are, it fits in with body typology rules. So, having learned this, you just have to learn to see it. This is the object of the next exercise.

Go to a place where you are likely to find people with a skin color that is different from your own. It could be a good reason to go out and enjoy a bowl of pasta in the Italian quarter or to take a walk in Chinatown. Do anything you like that allows you to watch a group of people with similar skin.

❖ First sit back and relax. Take a few deep breaths, setting aside all your usual worries for the moment. Clear your mind and concentrate on what you see.

❖ Look at the skin of the people around you. Do not worry if, because it is not like your own, the most striking thing about it at first is its shade. It is just that it is different from what you are used to. For the moment this does not matter. Keep working through the exercise.

❖ The first task, even if all these peoples' skin look the same to you, is to try and look for differences in complexion. Scan the faces, until one person's skin stands out from the rest. It may look a little redder, whiter, greener, or more yellow than the others! Do not yet try to classify this person's type but, for the moment, just observe what is distinctive. You are trying to gather information to acquire a reference color spectrum.

❖ Once you have been able to create a bank of colors to use as a reference, ask yourself whether this person is ample or angular. If it helps, you can cheat a little by referring back to the other physiological characteristics. Look at body shape and proportions. Study the shape of the face.

Have you been able to identify one or two people? Well done! Your perception is improving, which is all that matters for the moment.

Duration: 30 minutes

Exercise 12.

Finally—pulling it all together!

Now comes the exciting part! Seeing how the pieces all fit together. And it is going to be easier than you think, because of all those hours of observation you have behind you. You have been learning to observe a host of details that you never even used to notice.

In this exercise, you are going to need two or three friends, and you are going to invite them to an official morphological analysis session. Find a suitable spot where you will be free to observe, touch, compress, request a little more skin to be revealed and ask your questions undisturbed. Print out some evaluation forms from the website: antiagingthecure.com and use them for your notes, which will make the process easier.

- ❖ First, decide the subject's class (ample or angular) by observing the color palette, the predominant features of the face and especially the body shape.
- ❖ Observe the skin more closely—look at the arm and upper chest area.
- ❖ Pinch the skin to evaluate elasticity and the adhesion of the dermis and the epidermis.
- ❖ Press the skin to test capillary return and to check for possible infiltration of lymph.
- ❖ Ask the key questions.
- ❖ Compare what you observe to the predispositions of the types.

Remember that human beings are always more complex in reality than our theories would have us believe. It will probably happen that none of your friends is a pure-type. What we are attempting to do is not to stick labels on individuals, but to help them better understand their needs and particularities and to direct them towards a suitable preventive anti-aging therapy according to their predominant types.

Duration: 60 minutes

Conclusion: learn, take preventive action, maintain equilibrium

Anti-aging

As you have become familiar with type evaluations and learned about the different treatments I propose, you have come to understand the philosophy that underlies my approach: knowing ourselves, appreciating the ways in which we differ from each other and taking care of ourselves on a daily basis. The kind of beauty that will last over the years stems from prevention and starts at an early age. Other treatments, that are purely cosmetic, give a temporary boost—and this is not a bad thing, do not get me wrong—but my purpose in this book is to encourage you to consider a long-term preventive attitude. I hope that it has given you sufficient motivation to adopt and maintain the balanced approach. You certainly now have all the necessary tools at your disposal.

For me, health is expressed by the radiance of the skin, the flexibility of the joints, the vigor of a person's movements and the capacity to live in the present, in harmony both with oneself and with others. Of course, we can expect to evolve over time, and aging is just one of the factors in the process. The choices we make will either accelerate or slow down these changes.

Time always flows in the same direction. But, by choosing the right direction for our lives, we can considerably slow the appearance of signs of aging. By remaining ignorant, we speed up the aging process. We do have the means to combat ignorance; we do have what it takes to fight the onset of aging. Putting these techniques into effect can mean a completely new way of life. It is a question of working with nature instead of working against it.

Health is expressed by the radiance of the skin, the flexibility of the joints, the vigor of a person's movements and the capacity to live in the present, in harmony both with oneself and with others.

In this book, you have heard about Linda, Louise, Lynn and Jermaine. Though each of them was suffering from a different problem, they all had something in common–their lifestyle choices had created an imbalance, and none of them knew what their own body type was. Everything they did was contrary to their own natures. They were swimming against the current. They were exhausting themselves by doing things that went against who they were. They were struggling because they had never stopped to ask themselves that one important question, "Who am I?"

This is the same question that we asked ourselves as we once again recognize the value of ancient medicines. Whether we consider Greco-Roman, Chinese, or Ayurvedic medicine, we see an approach centered on the whole being of the individual. These medicines viewed illness as an outward manifestation of an energy imbalance and of inappropriate everyday lifestyle choices. They all started with the basic premise that human beings are not identical, and that different types emerge from this diversity.

The numerous observation exercises, questionnaires and case studies have taught you how to identify your dominant type. In all of the four areas that we have considered, i.e., skincare, nutrition, exercise and interpersonal relationships, you now have the means to make enlightened choices.

Through our exploration of typology, I am certain that I have been able to guide you towards a deeper knowledge of yourself and also a better understanding of your loved ones. Speaking personally, not one day goes by when typology does not help me understand the behavior, the values and the worries of those around me, either at home, with my family and friends, or with my colleagues at work. Equilibrium depends entirely on improving our knowledge of ourselves and of our environment.

Learn, take preventive action, maintain equilibrium

Learning, taking preventive action and maintaining equilibrium are the three processes that are the key to my whole approach. I truly hope that this book will be the springboard to revolutionizing the world of health and beauty. I hope, too, that it will make people see things from a different perspective. I would like to thank you for making this journey with me. Your future and your destiny are now in your own hands.

The future

My hope in writing this book was to help change and improve modern medicine. I anticipate that it will draw the attention of researchers, physicians of all branches of medicine, and pharmaceutical companies, and I hope that, in the future, they will be interested in incorporating my ideas into their work.

As for me, I will carry on with my intensive research. This book is only the first in a series. My intention is to continue my work, delving deeper into skincare as well as into the other areas that have been covered in the book. There is still a long way to go before we fully understand the differences between each of our bodies.

Hippocratic Oath

For over 2,000 years in Europe, and now throughout the western world, it has been the custom for doctors to swear the same oath that Hippocrates asked of his students.

Today, the "Hippocratic Oath," as it is known, has become little more than a ritual at the graduation ceremony. Many people do not know what it contains and, in practice, those doctors who do know what it is think of it only in terms of the moral requirement of confidentiality that is found in the last few lines.

I am going to quote the whole of the Hippocratic Oath to demonstrate how the doctor's role was perceived over 2,000 years ago in Greece.

I personally find particular inspiration in this passage of the oath: "I will apply dietetic measures for the benefit of the sick according to my ability and judgment; I will keep them from harm and injustice."

I would so much like to see a swing in modern medicine, a return towards those promises to "apply dietetic measures for the benefit of the sick," and "keep them from harm and injustice."

While, of course, letting people travel their own roads towards achieving their objectives.

> "I will apply dietetic measures for the benefit of the sick according to my ability and judgment; I will keep them from harm and injustice."

The oath

I swear by Apollo Physician and Asclepius and Hygieia and Panaceia and all the gods and goddesses, making them my witnesses, that

I will fulfill according to my ability and judgment this oath and this covenant:

To hold him who has taught me this art as equal to my parents and to live my life in partnership with him and, if he is in need of money, to give him a share of mine, and to regard his offspring as equal to my brothers in male lineage and to teach them this art—if they desire to learn it—without fee and covenant; to give a share of precepts and oral instruction and all the other learning to my sons and to the sons of him who has instructed me and to pupils who have signed the covenant and have taken an oath according to the medical law, but no one else.

I will apply dietetic measures for the benefit of the sick according to my ability and judgment; I will keep them from harm and injustice.

I will neither give a deadly drug to anybody who asked for it, nor will I make a suggestion to this effect. Similarly I will not give to a woman an abortive remedy. In purity and holiness I will guard my life and my art.

I will not use the knife, not even on sufferers from stone, but will withdraw in favor of such men as are engaged in this work.

Whatever houses I may visit, I will come for the benefit of the sick, remaining free of all intentional injustice, of all mischief and in particular of sexual relations with both female and male persons, be they free or slaves.

What I may see or hear in the course of the treatment or even outside of the treatment in regard to the life of men, which on no account one must spread abroad, I will keep to myself, holding such things shameful to be spoken about.

If I fulfill this oath and do not violate it, may it be granted to me to enjoy life and art, being honored with fame among all men for all time to come; if I transgress it and swear falsely, may the opposite of all this be my lot.

To my readers

If you have enjoyed reading the book and would like to comment, or if you have had any significant experiences that you would like to share, please write to me at: testimonials@manonpilon.com.

I encourage you to stay in touch! Subscribe on-line to my magazine by sending an e-mail to: testimonials@manonpilon.com, or visit the website: antiagingthecure.com, to access the latest information and advice on anti-aging.

Thanks to all of you!

Acknowledgements

I would like to thank my husband Amir, whose confidence and support have allowed me to realize my hopes and accomplish my dreams.

Thanks, also, to my three children, Samy, Adam and Sara, for their patience in not seeing quite as much of their mother as other children do. The sacrifices they have made are too numerous to mention, but, just by being there, they have supported me in all my projects. My wish for them is that they will grow up respecting their innermost natures, with a desire to get the best out of their personal strengths and weaknesses. This book is my gift to them.

Many thanks go to my babysitter, Pauline, and her husband, for taking care of my children as their own; this has allowed me to continue my research knowing that my children were safe in the excellent hands of two people who love them as much as I do.

Thank you to my parents who always encouraged me to develop my full potential and gave me the means to fulfill my dreams. I thank them for their support.

To my godmother and godfather, Julienne and André, I offer thanks for your encouragement. Many thanks also go to my aunts and uncles for their advice.

And I also want to thank my team, Europe Cosmétiques, EuropeLab and Platinum Equipment for their support, hard work and patience. I know it is not always easy to keep up with me, but thanks for always being there. I could not have done it without you all.

I would like to thank Bernard, for the interest he has shown in what was a completely new subject for him. His desire to understand has allowed this book to happen. Thank you to my publisher, Sgräff, to Isabelle, who saw and believed in my potential as a writer, and to her associate, Claude, for his unfailing encouragement, support and hard work. Thank you, also, to the entire production team.

I would also like to mention and thank Dr. Arie Benchetrit, Dr. Albert Benahïme, Dr. Jocelyne Genest and Dr. Lisa Lasher, among many others, for their friendly and professional support and for agreeing to reread my manuscript. This book has been enriched by their comments.

Thank you to all the doctors who have attended my workshops and conferences and thanks to all of you for asking many excellent questions. They have pushed me to continue my research and to make new discoveries.

It was always my dream to work in the field of beauty and health. If I have had the honor of being able to take part in the birth of medical spas in North America and around the globe, it was with the support of the many doctors and surgeons who want their patients to be able to experience personal transformations under the best possible conditions.

I would like to thank the owners of the spas and aesthetic clinics, as well as the estheticians themselves, who trusted in my recommendations of equipment and product lines. Together, we observed the clinical results that have given them confidence and rewarded me with their ongoing trust.

Thanks to my clients, all the people who have come to me for aesthetic treatment. They have shown me that, though my services are the first step towards the results they desire, their well-being and health are acquired through their own active efforts. They have been the ones to show me that the four body types (*red ovals, green squares, yellow rectangles* and *white circles*) reside in all humans, regardless of ethic origin, sex, or age.

They have allowed me to see how physical traits are transmitted from generation to generation, and how psychological and spiritual characteristics develop. Through them, I have understood the constraints linked to phenotype and the freedom associated with genotype. They have offered me the privilege of encouraging them in the constant quest for equilibrium that constitutes health.

I will finish by thanking all the people who, in their own ways, have assisted in the writing of this book and who have enabled me to continue learning throughout my 22-year journey in the field of aesthetics.

Bibliography

ABRAVANEL, Elliot D. *Dr. Abravanel's Body Type Diet and Lifetime Nutrition Plan.* New York: Bantam,1999.

ARNDT, Kenneth A., Philip E. LEBOIT, June K. ROBINSON and Bruce U. WINTROUB. *Cutaneous Medicine and Surgery, an Integrated Program in Dermatology,* Volume 1 and 2, Philadelphia: W. B. Sanders Company, 1996.

CARTON, Paul. *Diagnostic et conduite des tempéraments.* Paris: Librairie Le François, 1961.

CARTON, Paul. *Les clefs du diagnostic de l'individualité.* Brévannes: Paul Carton éditeur,1942.

CHEVALLIER, Andrew. *Encyclopedia of Medicinal Plants.* Montreal: Reader's Digest Selection, 1996.

CHILDRE, Doc. *One minute stress management,* 2nd ed. Boulder Creek, CA: Planetary Publications, 1998.

CHOPRA, Deepak. *Perfect Health.* Michigan: Three Rivers Press, 1999.

CROOK, William G. *The yeast connection,* New York: Random House, 1983.

GOLDMAN, MITCHEL P., ROBERT A. WEISS, JOHN J. BERGAN, EDS. *Varicose Veins and Telangiectasis,* 2nd ed. St. Louis, Missouri: Quality Medical Publishing, 1999.

HYMAN, Mark and Mark LIPONIS. *Ultra Prevention.* New York: Atria Books, 2003.

JACKOWSKI, Edward J. *Escape Your Shape.* New York: Simon & Schuster, 2001.

JENSEN, Karen and Lorna VANDERHAEGHE. *No More HRT: Menopause Treat the Cause,* Hillsburg, Ontario: Act Natural Corporation, 2002.

KIEFFER, Daniel. *Guide personnel des bilans de santé.* Éditions Jacques Granger éditeur, 1997.

KLATZ, Ronald. *Ten weeks to a Younger You.* Chicago, IL: Anti-Aging Industry, 1999.

KLATZ, Ronald and Robert GOLDMAN. *Stopping the clock: longevity for the new millenium,* 2nd ed. North Bergen, NJ: Basic Health Publications, 2002.

LAADING, Isabelle. *Les cinq saisons de l'énergie* Méolans-Revel: Éditions DesIris, 1998.

MASUNAGA, Shizuto. *Zen Shiatsu.* Paris: Guy Trédaniel and Éditions de la Maisnie, 1985.

MINDELL, Earl. *Vitamin Bible for the 21st century.* New York: Warner Books, 1999.

MURRAY, Michael and Joseph Pizzorno, *Encyclopedia of Natural Medicine,* 2nd ed. Rocklin, CA: Prime Health, 1998.

OHASHI, Vaturu. *Comprendre le langage du corps.* Paris: Guy Trédaniel and Éditions de la Maisnie, 1991.

RASSNER, Gernot. *Atlas of Dermatology,* 3rd ed. Media, PA: Williams & Wilkins, 1994.

REAVLEY, Nicola. *New Encyclopedia, Vitamins, Minerals, Supplements and Herbs.* New York, Bookman Press, 1998.

SEARS, Barry. *The Anti-Aging Zone.* New York, Regan Books, 1998.

SERVAN-SCHREIBER, David. *The Instinct to Heal.* New York: Rodale Press, 2004.

ULLIS, Karlis et Greg PTACEK. *Age Right : Turn Back the Clock With a Proven, Personnalized Antiaging Program.* New York, Simon & Schuster, 1999.

WEISS, Robert A. *Vein Diagnosis and Treatment.* New York: Mc Graw Hill, 2001.

WOLCOTT, William and Fahey TRISH, *The Metabolic Typing Diet,* New York: Doubleday, 2000.

Glossary

Alipidic (skin): dry skin lacking in oil.

Alpha hydroxy acid: chemical component that acidifies the skin or any product with a low pH and, in doing so, encourages exfoliation and stimulates mitosis (cell division). The most common alpha hydroxy acids are glycolic (often found in sugar cane), lactic, malic, tartaric and citric acid.

Alpha-lipoic acid (ALA): an antioxidant 400 times more powerful than vitamin C. Soluble in oil and water. Provides complete protection for cells and genetic material. In addition, it also stimulates cellular metabolism. Facilitates the recycling of vitamins C and E. Numerous clinical studies on the effects of alpha-lipoic acid have proven its role in diminishing the symptoms of diabetes. In Germany, doctors use alpha-lipoic acid as a supplement in the treatment of the first stages of diabetes. The prescribed dosage is 800 mg per day. Alpha-lipoic acid is one of the rare substances that can cross the blood-brain barrier to reach the brain cells, where protection is most needed. In fact, it has been shown that nutraceuticals rich in ALA reach the brain by way of the blood and increase production of glutathione in the brain, which in turn increases protection against the damage caused by free radicals. Low levels of glutathione have been linked to diseases like Alzheimer's, Parkinson's and other degenerative diseases of the brain. Glutathione also provides benefits relating to diabetes and weight loss, as it increases the elimination of glucose in the blood. This glucose is used in the production of energy, or ATP (adenosine triphosphate), indispensable and vital to the human organism and cellular renewal. Used to treat cardiac diseases and to help reduce the risk of heart attacks. Beneficial for cataracts and the protection of the retina.

Anti-inflammatory: any substance that controls inflammation such as the reddening of the surface or the underlying layers of the skin due to infection, bacteria, pH imbalance, or nutritional imbalance, etc.

Antioxidant: any substance that neutralizes free radicals. The human body produces its own natural antioxidants, but sometimes these are not sufficient to stabilize all the free radicals produced by oxidation. The body is then said to be experiencing "oxidative stress" (see free radicals).

Arteriosclerosis: fibrosis of arterial tissue that causes a hardening or thickening of the artery walls. Green squares and yellow rectangles are predisposed to arteriosclerosis. The result is a poor exchange of nutrients, gases, water and waste through the arterial walls.

Arthritis: acute inflammation of the joints caused, particularly, by deposits of uric acid crystals (gout), or calcium salts. This problem is common to white circles.

Atherosclerosis: formation of blood clots (LDL cholesterol) that obstruct blood circulation. Red ovals and white circles are predisposed to atherosclerosis.

Autonomic nervous system: includes both the sympathetic and parasympathetic nervous systems. It is called 'autonomic' because it acts alone and involuntarily. It regulates basic parameters of the body such as temperature, blood pressure, level of sugar in the blood and the pH of different fluids. It also triggers instinctive reactions such as the desire to sleep, to eat, to have sex, or to drink. Acting faster than conscious thought, this system decides whether a person will flee or attack (the so-called flight or fight response). The two parts of the autonomic system are always trying to strike the right balance. White circles tend to call upon their parasympathetic nervous systems. White circles, for instance, sleep easily after a large meal. They often lack muscle tone and are very loose in their joints. In green squares and yellow rectangles it is the sympathetic nervous system that is most called upon. Such people are often worried and stressed and tend to have stiff muscles.

Basal layer: the deepest layer of the epidermis. Responsible for pigmentation of the skin and cellular regeneration.

Bioflavonoids: contain a high concentration of hesperidin. Bioflavanoids are powerful antioxidants with antibacterial, antiviral, anti-inflammatory and antiallergenic properties.

Capillary: any microscopic or barely visible blood vessel located on the surface of the skin. These are the blood vessels that are visible on the face in cases of couperose (telangiectasia), the second stage of rosacea. They can also appear on the surface of the legs.

Cell: the basic unit of living tissue, made up of a nucleus and several organelles suspended in cytoplasm. Metabolic exchanges take place in the cell.

Central nervous system: this includes the brain (which sends out nervous impulses) and the spinal cord.

Cholesterol: a substance found among the lipids in the blood. It is useful and essential. It plays a role in the production of certain hormones as well as of cell membranes. Too much cholesterol in the blood can be dangerous for the arteries, in particular for the coronary arteries that nourish the fibers of the myocardium or heart muscle. Cholesterol is insoluble in blood. It is carried to the cells in proteins (called lipoproteins), of which the two most common are low-density lipoproteins (LDL) and high-density lipoproteins (HDL). When the level of LDL in the blood is too high, it forms fatty deposits, known as plaque or atheroma (see Atherosclerosis). This is why we call LDL "bad" cholesterol, while HDL is known as "good" cholesterol. In fact, both are beneficial to the body; it is an excess of LDL that is "bad."

Coenzyme Q10: coenzymes are substances that enzymes depend upon to function. Coenzyme Q10 works with three complex enzymes in the production and storage of energy in mitochondria. It is synthesized by the body and found in the blood as well as in the tissues. It is soluble in lipids. Taken as a dietary supplement, its antioxidant properties make it beneficial to red ovals in particular.

Collagen: a protein that gives skin its elasticity. When we do not have enough collagen, wrinkles start to appear. Collagen production begins to decline before the age of thirty. It is destroyed by the sun, smoking, air pollution, etc. Lack of collagen is a problem for the aging green square or yellow rectangle. There are both internal and external methods of stimulating the production of collagen. Among the external approaches are intense pulsed light and LED red light therapies, which stimulate fibroblasts (skin cells that produce collagen).

Connective tissue: white fibrous tissue surrounding muscles and supporting the dermis.

Copper: essential in the production of elastin and collagen, as well as for healthy skin, bones and joints. Ensures a uniform pigmentation of hair and skin (converts tyrosine into a usable state). Necessary for the conversion of iron into hemoglobin and, consequently, provides energy by facilitating iron absorption.

Cystic acne: sub-cutaneous infection that causes bumps on the skin. Pus is not visible.

Dandelion root: the dandelion has long been used in traditional medicine to stimulate the workings of the digestive and urinary systems. The potassium found in dandelion reinforces muscles and stabilizes sugar concentration. Dandelion root is a valuable source of organic sodium, used to ease ulcers, stomach problems and stiffness in the joints and muscles. These roots, it is claimed, also drain the kidneys and liver. Thanks to their diuretic and depurative action they help eliminate uric acid and hence are used in treating rheumatism and gallstones. Dandelion is an excellent blood purifier, and the vitamins and minerals it contains make it a marvelous spring tonic.

Dermis: the second layer of the skin. Vascularized by the circulatory and lymphatic systems. Contains fibroblasts, hair follicles and sweat glands, among other things. The dermis has several functions including oxygenation, elimination of water and toxins through sweat and providing skin strength and resilience. It is therefore responsible for the overall good health and appearance of the skin.

Elastin: a protein found in the dermis. Responsible for elasticity (firmness) and for the juncture between the epidermis and the dermis.

Epidermis: the outermost layer of the skin responsible for the protection of the body. The epidermis is what gives skin its texture and appearance. It is in this layer that wrinkles, pimples and all other slight imperfections such as scars, stretch marks, and areas of skin discoloration appear.

Exfoliation: the removal or peeling of the loose or partly-loose skin cells on the surface of the epidermis. Keratinocytes and corneocytes present on the surface may be affected, but can be replaced. After exfoliation, skin tone becomes lighter and the pores appear tighter. Skin texture is improved. Healthy facial skin should be exfoliated every 28 to 35 days by microabraison or by a gentle exfoliant, depending on the condition of the skin. Red ovals and white circles require less exfoliation than green squares and yellow rectangles.

Fibroblast: a cell responsible for the production of elastin and collagen. It forms the structural support of the skin. Yellow rectangles and green squares have less fibroblast production and consequently are more prone to wrinkles. Can be responsible for other conditions such as osteoarthritis.

Folic acid: gives the skin a pleasing appearance and a radiant complexion. Important for a healthy pregnancy. Reduces the risk of birth defects. Good supplement for arthritis. Anemia: plays an important role in the production of red and white blood cells. Reduces the risk of cardiovascular diseases.

Free radicals: these are produced within the body by oxidation, the same process that occurs when a metal rusts, an oil goes rancid, or a cream thickens and changes color. In moving, an oxygen atom can lose one of its peripheral electrons. The atom, now unstable, moves within the body looking for a free electron or for an atom from which it can, in turn, extract an electron. This unstable atom, which is missing an electron, is known as a free radical. We usually speak of them in the plural, since at any moment there are billions of them wandering through our bodies. They are one of the causes of the aging of the human body, due to the micro lesions they produce as they pass through internal cells.

Gommage: a gentle form of exfoliation that consists of one topical application of an exfoliant product (see Exfoliation).

Heart failure: a weakness in the heart muscle or valves that causes impaired blood circulation resulting in the risk of heart attack.

Hemoglobin: the substance in red blood cells that carries oxygen. Hemoglobin comprises a pigment called heme (containing iron atoms that give blood and, by extension, skin its red color), and a protein called globin. Oxygen molecules in the lungs pass through the bronchial walls into to the blood plasma and then penetrate the red blood cells where they link up with the iron molecules in the hemoglobin.

One hemoglobin molecule can take on four oxygen molecules.

Hydrolipic balance: the epidermis is best able to protect the body from the external environment when the hydrolipic balance is properly maintained. To ensure this balance, two conditions must co-exist: a sufficient quantity of water must be present and, in addition, the combination of sugars, lipids and proteins in the water must be balanced. Most agents that are too acid (such as alcohol) disrupt this moisture balance, causing the skin to appear dry, rough and cracked when the skin is not sufficiently hydrated, and waxy and oily when the combination with water does not occur properly. They often accentuate the fact that an imbalance exists in the activity of the sebaceous glands, which are responsible for the production of oil on the skin.

Hydrostatic pressure: assures the exchange of liquids between the blood and lymphatic circulatory systems, and the tissues. An excess of hydrostatic pressure provokes edema (swelling). External pressure can compensate for low hydrostatic pressure (see Pressotherapy).

Hypodermis: the third layer of skin under the dermis, made up of adipose cells. Its role is to protect and it helps to maintain body temperature.

Immune system: a system for defense against pathogenic agents such as viruses and bacteria that have penetrated the body. The immune system is made up of diverse cells and molecules that patrol the entire body and destroy anything they find that they cannot identify as belonging to the body. The main cells involved in the immune system are lymphocytes, macrophages and dendrite cells. The immune system is very effective against metastatic cancerous cells. More than 99% of the cells that circulate with the blood or lymphatic circulatory systems are destroyed before they can find a place at which to settle and develop a new tumor. The skin and mucosa help the immune system by presenting a barrier to the entry of foreign microorganisms.

Inflammatory acne: development of bacteria in the follicles or pores, which causes pimples (with or without pus) or comedons (blackheads) on the skin.

Integument: everything that grows at the periphery of the body, including hair, eyelashes, nails and teeth. Its principal component is keratin.

Laser: a device that uses resonance to produce amplified wavelengths of monochromatic light. Lasers can be blue, green, yellow and red, among others. Some skin treatments use a particular type of laser. For example, in cases of skin badly damaged by the sun, doctors use a carbon dioxide (CO_2) laser to resurface (peel) the skin to reveal the new skin underneath. This treatment, however, is not without pain. The skin takes three months to stabilize. A Nd: YAG laser is used to remove hair and varicose veins, while a Q-switch laser is used to remove tattoos.

L-cysteine: (n-acetyl-cysteine) participates in numerous metabolic activities (synthesis of fatty acids; production of skin, nails and hair; production of hormones; etc.). In particular, it is needed to synthesize glutathione (an important antioxidant) and to maintain the required amount in the cells. L-cysteine helps prevent the damaging oxidation of ascorbic acid and polyunsaturated fatty acids. It also protects the body from radiation and oxidative stress.

LED: the acronym for Light-Emitting Diode. A device that emits light of a determined wavelength and, hence, color. The depth to which the light beams will penetrate the skin varies depending on the selected color. Different conditions can be treated depending on the skin layer reached (epidermis, dermis). For example, to stimulate the production of collagen by fibroblasts located in the dermis, a red light beam at a wavelength of 640 nanometers is used. Acne is treated with a blue beam at a wavelength of between 400 and 470 nanometers; pigment spots or redness are treated with a green beam at a wavelength of around 525 nanometers.

Licorice root: licorice has many medicinal properties. It has been used for thousands of years to treat urinary and gastrointestinal problems. It has a therapeutically calming and protective effect on the adrenal glands. Licorice softens the skin and acts as an anti-inflammatory agent. Recent studies have shown that licorice has a rejuvenating effect on the cells of the digestive system, a remarkable effect on the liver, and can also act as an antioxidant within the body. These studies also showed the beneficial effects of licorice in cases of cancer and of arthritis.

Lipid: pertaining to lipids. Fat. (See Hydrolipic balance.)

Lymph: as interstitial liquid enters the lymphatic vessels, it is called lymph (from the Latin word lympha meaning water). Only the name changes; its principal composition remains the same. It contains water, mineral salts, waste products, pathogens, proteins and white blood cells. Lymph is more viscous than water.

Lymphatic drainage: one of the techniques used in massotherapy, lymphatic drainage is a way of improving circulation throughout the lymphatic system. In this way, it also facilitates the elimination of wastes and toxins by the macrophages (white blood cells), as it pushes the lymph towards the lymph nodes where this transformation occurs.

Magnolia vine: most studies claim that magnolia has a beneficial effect on diseases related to hepatitis. The lignins of the berry protect the liver by stimulating anti-oxidizing cells. Magnolia is considered to be a medicinal plant because of its exceptional effects, which are similar to those of ginseng: regulation of the central nervous system, cerebral stimulation and improved reflexes and endurance.

Melanin: a pigment found in the top layer of the skin, in the eyes, eyelashes and hair. Melanin is responsible for skin color and, when an imbalance occurs, for hyperpigmentation of the skin: melasma, patches of facial discoloration, brown marks in pregnancy known as chloasma, or liver spots (also known as age spots).

Mesotherapy: injection of a fat-reducing solution to reduce unattractive fat buildup. Can improve body contours, but is not a solution to obesity or cellulite.

Metabolism: the fundamental biochemical process of the human body that occurs in each cell. It is summarized by this equation: nutrients + O_2 = energy (ATP) +water + heat + waste + CO_2. The nutrients and oxygen carried by the blood are delivered by the capillaries and enter the cells. Millions of chemical reactions take place in the cells at the same time. The end products: energy, stored as ATP (adenosine triphosphate) in the mitochondria; heat; water; carbon dioxide; and waste products that are transported by blood or lymph, then transformed and eliminated.

Microdermabrasion: mechanical exfoliation of the epidermis performed by a specialized apparatus.

Minerals: zinc, iron, copper, magnesium, calcium, silicon and chromium are all minerals that catalyze metabolic reactions in cells. These minerals are found in vegetables, fruits, mineral water and food supplements. Certain vitamins such as vitamins B and E are not absorbed if sufficient quantities of certain minerals are not present in the body.

Mitochondria: small components of cells that provide energy to the cell. Very active cells such as those of muscle fibers have many mitochondria. Less active cells such as white blood cells only have a few mitochondria. When the body's needs for energy increase, mitochondria can reproduce so as to be able to meet the increased demand. Mitochondria also affect your genetic material as they contain DNA.

Mitosis: the continual process in which the nucleus of a living cell divides to form two daughter cells.

Moisturizer: any product that helps to maintain the skin's hydrolipic balance. Wherever applied, its oil component retains moisture in the skin.

Morpho-lympho drainage: a manual technique developed in Switzerland and forming part of the Physiodermie skincare method. It consists of a rapid and effective drainage of the face (in 8 minutes) or of the entire body (in 20 minutes). It includes morpho-digestive massage, which consists of brushing, kneading and vibrating the colon.

Non-inflammatory acne: well-known symptoms are open comedons (blackheads) and closed comedons (whiteheads).

Omega-3, -6 and -9: help slow arteriosclerosis. Reduce the level of LDL cholesterol and of triglycerides. Reduce the viscosity of the blood and help prevent heart attacks. Preserve the health of the skin, nails and hair. Help reduce high blood pressure. Improve the effectiveness of the immune system. Alleviate the symptoms of arthritis and of rheumatoid arthritis. Help ease migraines. Help alleviate kidney diseases. Unsaturated fatty acids of types omega-3, -6 and -9 are indispensable for keeping the skin supple and soft and the complexion clear. As we age, our bodies stop making enough essential fatty acids (EFAs) to maintain good hydration and nutrition of the skin cells.

Osteoarthritis: the wear and tear of cartilage and inadequate elasticity of the supporting tissue. Most often found in green squares and yellow rectangles.

Parasympathetic nervous system: associated with rest, relaxation, digestion and slowing down the heart rate.

Peeling: deep exfoliation by means of chemical substances or mechanical action.

Pendulum: excrescence of the skin fed by arterial and venous capillaries. Pendulums can be removed by electrocoagulation.

pH: the pH of pure water is 7. This is the neutral point between acidity and alkalinity. The pH of healthy skin is 5.5, more acid than pure water. Blood has a pH of around 7.5. It is more alkaline than water. Measurements of pH indicate the relative acidity of a skincare product, a liquid or cellular tissue at a specific moment. Is it more acidic than normal? More alkaline?

Pressotherapy: a technique using compression boots to facilitate venous and lymphatic circulation. Helpful for people with edema in the legs, hydric cellulite, venous insufficiency, or venous ulcers.

Red blood cell: a blood cell that has no nucleus. Transports oxygen in the arteries and carbon dioxide in the veins. Essential for healthy skin and other tissues of the body.

Rosacea: a neurovascular imbalance that provokes a chronic cutaneous condition appearing on the face as redness, first intermittent and later permanent. This is not a simple problem of the complexion, but a disease whose symptoms can be alleviated by laser treatments, IPL, electrocoagulation or sclerotherapy. Acne rosacea is commonly known as blotchiness. It is caused by proliferation of Demodex folliculorum, a microscopic mite. The evolution of rosacea develops in 5 stages:

1. Diffuse redness
2. Telangiectasia (couperose)
3. Acne rosacea
4. Rhinophyma
5. Ocular rosacea

Silymarin: extracted from the seeds of the plant called Silybum marianum or milk thistle, frequently used to treat liver diseases. It helps prevent liver diseases due to alcohol abuse, drugs, the oxidative effects of pesticides and poisons, and hepatitis. The active ingredients in milk thistle are what are known as flavonoids. The specific flavonoids in milk thistle are silybin, silydianin and silychristin, collectively known as silymarin. Milk thistle is a remarkable herb. It has been proven that it can protect the liver from numerous stresses, such as the harmful effects of environmental toxins, alcohol, drugs and chemotherapy. Silybin, one of the active chemical components of the plant, functions as an antioxidant and as one of the most potent liver-protecting agents known. Clinical tests have proven silybin to be effective in treating chronic liver diseases in protecting the liver from toxic chemical products.

Sympathetic nervous system: makes the body react to an alarm by, for instance, producing adrenalin, increasing the heart rate and stimulating intense muscle activity (flight or fight).

Telangiectasia (couperose): characterized by the appearance of superficial and dilated violet venules or red arterioles on the face, often called spider veins or blotches.

Topical: topical products are applied directly to the skin. Examples include creams, serums, tonics and lotions.

UVA: ultraviolet rays emitted by the sun at wavelengths between 400 and 320 nanometers.

UVB: ultraviolet rays emitted by the sun at wavelengths between 320 and 290 nanometers.

Varicose vein: vein with a dilated wall, forming a visible pocket on the leg. The vein may clearly increase in diameter and stick out like a strand of spaghetti. Varicose veins may also be due to a malfunction of the vein wall so that it is too permeable, or a failure of the valve in the vein, causing it to remain too open or too closed. Sometimes, surgery is required to remove varicose veins.

Varicosity: venous insufficiency. Dilated capillaries visible on the surface of the skin, usually on the legs, forming what are called spider veins (see Telangiectasia).

Vasoconstrictor: any product that reduces the diameter of a blood or a lymph vessel is called a vasoconstrictor.

Vasodilator: any product that enlarges the diameter of a blood or a lymph vessel is called a vasodilator.

Venous insufficiency: a weakness in the long and short saphenous veins (in the legs), resulting in poor drainage of venous blood back to the heart. This imbalance in the flow of blood to and from the heart results in varicose veins, telangiectasia, or swelling of the surrounding tissue, even producing dry skin and vascular ulcers.

Vitamin A: the name given to a group of oil-soluble components such as carotene. Vitamin A helps the body by, among other things, protecting it from infections and attacks by microorganisms; it is used, for example, in acne treatments. It is also an antioxidant that acts against oil-soluble free radicals. It is also necessary for the formation of collagen. Vitamin A is found in, among other sources, liver, whole milk and egg yolks. The intestine absorbs it in the presence of lipids. It becomes toxic in very large quantities.

Vitamin B: the name given to a group of water-soluble components of which the best known are thiamin (B1), riboflavin (B2), folic acid, biotin and vitamin B12. Vitamin B plays a wide variety of roles. For instance, it affects the nervous system, the metabolism and the health of certain tissues such as the skin, nails and hair. It is found in, among other sources, brown rice, liver, grains, nuts, eggs, beans and all green vegetables. Since it is never stored for long in the body, it should be taken regularly.

Vitamin B1: also known "the morale vitamin" because of its known benefits to the balance of the nervous system. The body better absorbs it when it is part of a B vitamin complex, especially in balanced combination with vitamins B2 and B6. It is important in maintaining the nervous system, muscles and heart in good working order. It is an important supplement for keeping and improving mental functions and concentration in alcoholics and in the elderly. It helps digestion, particularly of carbohydrates (sugars). It stimulates the growth of skin cells and of the organism in general. It helps in treating herpes. It has no known toxic effects. But watch out! Caffeine, alcohol and acidic or processed foods are enemies of vitamin B1 and prevent the body from assimilating it.

Vitamin B12: (cobalamin). Because vitamin B12 needs calcium to be well absorbed by the stomach, we recommend taking it with calcium-rich foods such as milk, cheese, tofu, salmon, peanuts, nuts, broccoli and soybeans. Vitamin B12 is involved in a large number of important metabolic processes, including the synthesis of DNA, the formation of blood cells, and the maintenance of the heart and nervous system in good health. Helps attenuate brown spots or hyperpigmentation. It is known as "the red vitamin" because it contributes to the formation of red blood cells. It is an important supplement for treating anemia. Recommended as a supplement for depression, neurological problems and insomnia. It keeps the nervous system balanced and eases irritability. Beneficial before and during menstruation. Helps with memory and concentration. Essential for the elderly and those suffering from Alzheimer's disease. Boosts energy. Helps prevent cancer induced by cigarette smoking.

Vitamin B2: because they eat a poorly balanced diet, the majority of North Americans suffer from a lack of vitamin B2. It is beneficial for the health of the skin, nails and hair, and helps prevent hair loss. It is indispensable for good vision because it helps the eyes relax. It helps in treating cataracts. It helps ease the pain of sore lips or tongue. It is a good supplement for dealing with arthritis, carpal tunnel syndrome and migraine. If you drink too much alcohol, it will be difficult for your body to absorb vitamin B2.

Vitamin B3: (niacinamide). Restores good health and a relaxed tone to your skin. Needed for the good health of the digestive system, it alleviates gastrointestinal troubles. It helps reduce high blood pressure, cholesterol and triglycerides. Alleviates bad breath. If your skin is sensitive to the sun, you might be lacking vitamin B3. Beneficial for migraine and arthritis.

Vitamin B5: (pantothenic acid). Improves the responses of the immune system and the production of antibodies for fighting infections. Helps reduce high levels of cholesterol and triglycerides in the blood. Intervenes in the transformation of lipids and sugars into energy. Vitamin B5 is vital for the proper functioning of the adrenal glands and for maintaining hormonal equilibrium. Helps wounds heal. Helps the growth and development of nervous system cells. Vitamin B5 is very helpful in treating postoperative shock, fatigue and allergies.

Vitamin B6: (pyridoxine). Necessary for the absorption of vitamin B12 and for maintaining the proper level of magnesium in the body. Helps prevent skin imperfections such as eczema, psoriasis and dermatitis. Necessary for healthy hair. Helps calm irritability and anxiety due to menstruation. Helps prevent kidney stones.

Vitamin C: involved in more than 100 biological processes in the body. Plays an essential role in the production of collagen and adrenalin, and as an antioxidant in the fight against free radicals. Soluble in water. Found in fruits and vegetables. It is absorbed in the intestine, and the urine eliminates any excess within two or three hours. When adding it to the diet in the form of supplements, therefore, one should not take huge doses at one time, but rather doses of 500 mg spaced out over time.

Vitamin E: the name given to a complex of components (tocopherol and tocotrienol) that are oil-soluble. Its main role is as a powerful antioxidant. It is found in nuts and grains, cereals and green vegetables. Absorbed in the intestine and the liver in the presence of lipids and of bile. Vitamin E can also become very toxic if it is not in the right form or if taken in too large a quantity.

Vitamin H: (biotin), considered to be part of the B vitamin group. Vitamin H plays a role as a co-enzyme in the metabolism of proteins, carbohydrates and lipids. Plays an important role in preventing hair loss. Limits the appearance of gray hair. An important supplement for preventing fragile nails from breaking or crumbling. Eases muscle pain. Helps to sooth eczema and dermatosis (skin disease). Biotin is more effective when combined with vitamin B2, B6 and B3; all these vitamins act together synergistically. A biotin deficiency can cause serious problems with the immune system, nerves, muscles, hair and skin. This is because biotin forms part of several enzymes in our bodies that control such vital functions as the activity of white blood cells, the synthesis of proteins and fatty acids, and the metabolism of carbohydrates and sugars. All the B vitamins are water-soluble. An excess of these vitamins is not stored in the body, but easily eliminated through the urine.

White blood cell: an immune cell, active in the blood, cutaneous tissues and lymph nodes. White blood cells known as macrophages remove pathogens and debris (a combination of dead cells, proteins, lipids and sugars) that are carried by the lymph. In white circles, macrophages located in the lymph nodes are not efficient at filtering and removing this debris, as lymph reaches the nodes too slowly. In cutaneous tissue, this stagnation (edema) of lymph laden with waste and toxins can even become the cause of localized infection (acne).

Zinc: a vital oligo-element for several metabolic processes in our organism. Indispensable for the fabrication of collagen and for cellular renewal. Helps eliminate white spots on the nails. Serves as a component of several enzymes including superoxide dismutase (SOD), which acts as an antioxidant. Indispensable for the teeth, bones, nails, hair and skin. Also required for the proper functioning of the immune system. Contributes to ridding the organism of toxins such as alcohol. Helps healing.

List of exercises, questionnaires, boxes and games